The Cancer Breakthrough

A nutritional approach
for doctors and patients

Drs. Hickey and Roberts have been in the forefront of non-toxic cancer therapies. Their insights into various subjects, especially in the use of ascorbic acid in cancer therapy presented in their publications, are an important contribution and relevant in the understanding of its effectiveness. This new book is another valuable and needed contribution. The information put together in this book is not available elsewhere. It is a straightforward compendium of what to do when you have cancer, written for doctors and patients. Congratulations Drs. Hickey and Roberts for this contribution. We are very happy they are on our side. The dark side is not so dark any more.

Dr Jorge Miranda Massari
And
Dr Michael J. Gonzalez Guzman

ISBN 978-1-4303-2300-6

The Cancer Breakthrough

A nutritional handbook
for doctors and patients

by

Steve Hickey PhD

and

Hilary Roberts PhD

Acknowledgements

Our research into cancer has benefited from the cooperation of many scientists and physicians. In particular, we would like to thank Dr Abram Hoffer for his help and support. Dr Robert Cathcart generously shared his expertise in discussions with us on the properties of vitamin C. Bill Sardi sent us information about recent developments in nutrition and cancer. Dr Andrew Saul's encouragement was invaluable. Dr Damien Downing, of the British Society for Ecological Medicine, provided background data on the effects of Herceptin and other anticancer drugs. Further general support has been provided by Dr Olga Gregson, Professor Terry Looker and Professor Bill Gilmore.

The work of the late Dr Hugh Riordan provided scientific data for this book. His research group, RECNAC (cancer in reverse), and associates continue to do pioneering work. Particular thanks go to Dr Jorge Miranda Massari and Dr Michael Gonzalez, for their dedication to research into antioxidants and cancer. They reviewed a copy of this book before publication, giving us valuable feedback. Dr Mark Levine of the National Institutes of Health and his research team have recently replicated some of the work on vitamin C and cancer, providing increased media exposure for what is an underreported health story.

The popular media have not reported the story on vitamin C and cancer. In general, they do not report health matters fairly, providing support and publicity (some would say propaganda) for pharmaceutical companies and associated interests. Claims for vitamin C and other nutrients are ignored: a remarkable bias. Fortunately, some reporters, including Bill Sardi and Gaillon Totheroh, campaign for open reporting of nutrition and health. Owen Fonorow and the Vitamin C Foundation have continued to keep Linus Pauling's legacy in the public view.

Biolab Medical Unit, London, England, provided us with facilities for an experiment on blood levels of vitamin C in subjects with dynamic flow intakes of vitamin C. We would like to thank Biolab, London for their help and particularly Mark Howard, Dr Nicholas Miller, Melita Dean, Hannah Quirke and Christine Hemmingway.

Michael Roberts, FRCS, provided feedback and discussion on the approach of this and other of our texts. Dr Reginald Holman, a pioneer of redox approaches to cancer treatment, provided detailed comments and discussion of points, indicating where we had oversimplified biology or presentation. Dr Len Noriega kindly read the book and provided background comment.

Holly.Matthies and Andrew Hickey checked the text for accuracy and readability. Andrew also donated weeks of his time in the analysis of clinical trials of vitamin C and cancer, providing invaluable background for our understanding of the subject. Dr Nadia Roberts, Gillian Perkins and Stephanie Morgan kindly checked the text for errors, providing help with the presentation of a difficult subject.

Preface

Since publishing *Cancer: Nutrition and Survival*,[1] we have been asked repeatedly which nutritional supplements are most appropriate to treat, or prevent, cancer. The question is not straightforward, as relevant research is sparse compared to the number of potentially effective supplements. This book presents our current response to such requests. It was a subject we wished rather to avoid, as it relates directly to therapy. However, we decided that unless we were specific about the requirements, people might undertake clinical trials based on an inappropriate selection and dose of supplements and diet.

Poorly designed studies abound in the area of vitamin C. For example, a study of vitamin C which employed a single, daily, oral 10 gram dose would show little benefit, as the absorption would be limited and the excretion rate too high for a reasonable expectation of a pharmacological effect.

Cancer: Nutrition and Survival covers the background science, giving a new perspective on cancer as an evolutionary disease. We explain how the development, growth and survival of cancer cells are influenced by antioxidants and oxidants. The present book describes the implications of our microevolutionary model and suggests a nutritional protocol for cancer patients. The doses of supplements we suggest are appropriate for adults.

These suggestions are aimed at doctors and other professionals, who have the training and expertise to evaluate the programme and monitor patient progress. They are not intended for self-treatment. Treatment of serious diseases, such as cancer, requires the supervision of a qualified health care professional.

Books on cancer enter an emotive and combative arena. Vested interests abound, as the profits from cancer treatment are massive. In science generally, it is conventional to have an open exchange of ideas and data. In the health field, such discussion is gradually being degraded. Critics frequently claim that 'there is no scientific proof' that a treatment works. Such claims are themselves unscientific. Indeed, they are true for all science, as the scientific method does not enable proof.

---

[1] Hickey S. and Roberts H. (2005) Cancer: Nutrition and Survival, Lulu Press.

Science progresses quickly when the extent of our ignorance is understood and accepted. Proof, with its implication of absolute knowledge, has no place in science: it belongs to the realms of mathematics and logic. Science is the process of providing models of the world that fit with observations of reality. When a model, or theory, does not fit the facts, it is rejected.

Concepts such as 'medical proof', which purport to demonstrate absolute knowledge, inhibit future developments. A recent example of this is the time it took to establish an association between helicobacter pylori and stomach ulcers. Since many people believed it had been 'proved' that stress caused ulcers, they were slow to admit the possibility of an alternative explanation. Consequently, research showing an infectious origin was delayed. The idea that ulcers are associated with bacteria is now accepted, allowing treatment with antibiotics.

Our interpretation of demands for 'scientific proof' is that they stifle innovation, causing delays to research and evaluation. Nutritional supplements that could be of value in cancer require scientific testing, not to be brushed under the carpet by a demand for 'proof,' with no provision of funding for clinical trials. Cancer treatment is highly regulated but, when only the pharmaceutical industry can afford to comply, this regulation can act against the interest of patients. We are not promoting any particular product or therapy, but understand the frustration of scientists who are aware of evidence in favour of non-patentable agents, yet cannot access the funding for appropriate clinical trials.

The authors are not physicians and do not claim to be competent to treat patients: as scientists, our job is to explain the implications of research findings. The aim of this book is to inform and educate. Although we believe it is in the public interest for this information to be made widely available, we stress that anyone electing to follow the suggestions does so at their own risk. The authors cannot be held responsible for the use or misuse of this information.

We hope doctors will consider passing on the information to their patients and have written the book with this possibility in mind. The supporting scientific data is presented in *Cancer: Nutrition and Survival*, which contains more than a thousand scientific references. Readers wanting further information are directed to this source or the suggested reading in Appendix 3.

After reviewing the scientific evidence, we have come to the conclusion that it may be possible to control many cancers by dietary means. In particular, redox-active nutrients offer the promise of a safe anticancer therapy, which may be more effective than current chemotherapy. We therefore have no choice but to provide this information to practising physicians and scientists.

As with our other books, we invite doctors, scientists and other interested parties to email comments or errors to us at radicalascorbate@yahoo.com. This allows readers to act as reviewers of the text, helping to ensure that the contents are factually correct, or at least consistent with current scientific knowledge.

Contents

"Everyone should know that most cancer research is largely a fraud and that the major cancer research organisations are derelict in their duties to the people who support them."

Linus Pauling

The cancer wars

'The doctor of the future will give no medicine but will interest his patients in the care of the human frame, in diet and in the cause and prevention of disease.' Thomas Edison

Simple dietary changes can greatly increase the life expectancy of people with cancer. Redox therapy involves specific dietary supplements, which kill cancer cells or slow the growth of tumours while leaving healthy cells unharmed. This therapy can be enhanced by cutting down on calories, particularly sugars and starches - the favoured foods of cancer cells.

So why, if this cheap and simple way of controlling cancer is effective, is its use not commonplace? As one sceptical patient argued, 'If it worked, hospitals would already be giving it to patients.' This assertion assumes doctors already know everything about treating cancer which, unfortunately, is not the case. Cancer research is so complex and fragmented that physicians are unable to keep track of developments.

To understand why this promising therapy is not in everyday use, we need to examine the recent history of cancer treatment. In 1971, US President Richard Nixon declared war on cancer. He pledged 'an extra $100 million to launch an intensive campaign to find a cure'. Nonetheless, thirty-five years later, four out of every ten US citizens still get the disease at some point in their lives, and one in five die of it. Anyone whose friends or family have suffered from cancer will have experienced the pervasive fear of the disease and will know how difficult it can be to treat.

Over decades, scientists have made little progress in finding a cure, or even effective treatments. There has been reasonable improvement in treating some rare cancers, particularly those in childhood. However, the main killers are solid tumours, occurring later in life. These do not respond well to the therapies currently available to physicians.

You might find the previous paragraph surprising, as such claims are frequently contradicted in the media. Many people believe that treatments are improving all the time, as they read in the newspapers. They imagine that increased research spending will soon solve the problem. However, the long-awaited breakthrough, which politicians of the 1970s thought was just a few years away, remains elusive. Furthermore, media misinformation, far from being harmless, makes it difficult for cancer sufferers to benefit from findings that fall outside the mainstream.

Consider Herceptin, touted as 'the largest improvement in outcome for any group of women with breast cancer in 25 years'.[a] As a result of such wild claims, the media have been highlighting the plight of women who, they claim, will die unless they get the new wonder drug. Herceptin is not even as new as articles suggest: it was approved by the US FDA in September 1998, as a second or third line therapy for treatment of certain patients with last stage breast cancer.

Despite the hype, Herceptin provides only a marginal increase in survival compared to not taking it. The women highlighted by the media were apparently not told that Cancer Research UK have estimated the average life expectancy for people with early stage breast cancer is about 20 years. Taking an optimistic view, Herceptin will add only a few months to this, at the risk of heart failure and other side effects. If this is an 'astonishingly effective wonder drug,' then cancer therapy is in big trouble.

The cost of one year's treatment with Herceptin is of the order of 70,000 US dollars. In the UK, the Health Service is publicly urged to find the funds to provide such therapies. Other public health services, for example, in Ontario, Canada, have bowed to public pressure and agreed to pay for the drug, despite their doubts about its efficacy. Not surprisingly, several of these pressure groups are supported by the pharmaceutical industry.

There is no comparable campaign for drug companies to lower their exorbitant prices. Nor is there a popular movement to change the patent laws, to reduce excessive profits made at the expense of the sick, even though proceeds are disproportionate to the efforts companies make in supporting scientific research.[b,c] Those few reporters and doctors who have queried prices have been told that they are in line with research costs. Yet, when asked for a cost breakdown, the drug companies have refused to provide one.

The use of cytotoxic chemotherapy, or 'chemo', has increased, in terms of the quantity of available drugs and the number of patients using them. For some rare cancers, chemotherapy can extend life; it can even be curative. Unfortunately, it is futile for most adult cancers, though its

---

[a] Moss R.W. (2005) Herceptin or Deceptin, The Moss Reports, December 18.
[b] Angell M. (2004) The truth about the drug companies, Random House, New York.
[c] Goonzer M. (2004) The $800 million dollar pill, University of California Press, Berkley.

side effects can be devastating. Chemotherapy grew out of research into chemical weapons. Unlike penicillin, which kills an infection but does not harm the patient, chemo often injures the patient as much as it does the cancer.[d]

Most claims for chemotherapy are misleading. It provides an effective therapy, with greater than 10% increase in survival, for cancers of the cervix, testes, and for lymphomas. However, in 2004, three Australian cancer specialists stated that, 'The overall contribution of curative and adjuvant cytotoxic chemotherapy to 5-year survival in adults was estimated to be 2.3% in Australia and 2.1% in the USA.'[e] They added, 'As the 5-year relative survival rate for cancer in Australia is now over 60%, it is clear that cytotoxic chemotherapy only makes a minor contribution to cancer survival. To justify the continued funding and availability of drugs used in cytotoxic chemotherapy, a rigorous evaluation of the cost-effectiveness and impact on quality of life is urgently required.'

Health experts and the media have failed to report that, for most cancers, standard chemotherapy is only marginally effective. To achieve even this modest result, the side effects of conventional chemotherapy have become notoriously well known. The popular image of a pale, bald and nauseous cancer patient arises more from the effects of treatment, particularly chemotherapy, than the disease itself. Since the 1970s, the highly funded 'war on cancer' has been a resounding failure. Claims for improvements in conventional treatments have been over-hyped and reality does not reflect the popular myth.

Surprisingly, even before President Nixon's announcement of the war against cancer, scientists had discovered a non-poisonous form of chemotherapy. This was ignored by the mainstream, profit-driven effort to combat cancer. What followed was an under-funded guerrilla war, running in parallel with the conventional approach.

This smaller, though arguably more successful, campaign began with the isolation and identification of vitamin C, in 1932. Albert Szent-Gyorgyi, who received the Nobel Prize for his achievements, believed that people needed large amounts of vitamin C to prevent, and possibly treat, cancer. Only two years after vitamin C's identification, a chemist called Irwin Stone began investigating the properties of vitamin C. Stone

d Penicillin is less safe than commonly realised and can cause death from anaphylactic shock.
e Morgan G, Ward R, Barton M. (2004) The contribution of cytotoxic chemotherapy to 5-year survival in adult malignancies. Clin Oncol (R Coll Radiol), 16(8), 549-560.

also thought that people needed large doses to prevent and treat disease. Perhaps his greatest contribution was to get another Nobel laureate, Linus Pauling, interested in vitamin C.

Pauling, in collaboration with Scottish surgeon, Ewan Cameron, published results of clinical trials of vitamin C and cancer. Japanese researchers, Murata and Morishige, and, independently, Abram Hoffer, a Canadian physician, also published clinical studies on the effectiveness of vitamin C in the treatment of cancer. There was something odd about the results of these experiments: patients lived longer – much longer. Those treated with vitamin C lived an average of four times as long as control patients who did not receive vitamin C. This massive improvement was unparalleled in the history of medicine.

Selfish Cells

'It amazes me how much of what passes for knowledge in cancer therapy turns out to be incomplete, inadequate and anecdotal.' Ralph Moss.

The basic structural and functional unit of the human body is the cell. Within our bodies, microscopic cells are continually dividing and dying. For example, skin cells are constantly sloughed off and replaced; we lose about a gram of dead skin every day. What we do affects how our skin responds: the skin on our palms and soles can thicken to form calluses, in response to the applied stresses of working or walking. Despite shedding cells, the process of skin growth and death is highly controlled. Apart from age-related changes, skin retains its overall form for many years.

Bodily tissues (groups of cells with similar functions) are continually repaired and replaced. Over a period of years, most of the molecules that make up our tissues are replaced by others from the diet. The statement, 'we are what we eat,' is true. Even something as apparently inert as bone is a dynamic, biological system, with new bone being formed as old bone is destroyed.

A correct balance between production of new cells and death of old ones is essential to health. For example, if new bone is created more slowly than old bone is destroyed, then osteoporosis, a disease characterised by weak, thinning bones, can result. Conversely, cells that multiply more quickly than old ones are destroyed may become a tumour. The control of cell growth and death is critical to our well-being. Cell number is highly controlled, by a complex arrangement of signals.

Occasionally, some cells break free of their normal growth controls, to become cancerous. Cancer cells can divide at a higher rate than healthy cells and can ignore the signals that tell normal cells to die. The result is an abnormal growth of tissue.

Cells commit suicide

So that our tissues can remain in good condition, cells need to be able to die when they are no longer needed. This allows them to be replaced by fresh, healthy cells. To do this, cells have an inbuilt mechanism for cell suicide; this is called *apoptosis*.

At the start of apoptosis, a cell receives specific signals that instruct it to kill itself. In response, it goes through a controlled process, during which it shuts down and dies. It is important that these signals are clear and unambiguous: otherwise, cells could misinterpret them and die unnecessarily.

It may seem strange that cells should commit suicide, but this controlled cell death is an essential feature of multicellular organisms, such as animals and plants. Take the process of forming structured organs, during a baby's development. Hands, for example, begin as mitten-like protuberances, but then the cells between what will become fingers die, to leave fully-formed hands.

We witness many examples of programmed cell death; perhaps most dramatic is when the autumn leaves of deciduous trees wither and fall, to be renewed each spring. This loss of leaves could be advantageous to the tree, allowing it to rest during the winter, or to shed parasites with the dead tissue.

Bacteria

Bacteria are small, single-celled life forms: each cell is an independent organism. A typical bacterium is tiny: about a thousandth of a millimetre long. This means that they can be spread by touch or even by air currents. Some cause illnesses, such as sore throats; others are beneficial, including the 'friendly bacteria,' in our guts. In a receptive environment, with a source of food, bacteria can grow rapidly. A single cell can start a colony of billions, by growing larger and splitting into two. These offspring cells are identical to the original and can each divide, repeatedly, to produce others.

Bacteria are essential to life on earth. They break down dead animals and plants, making their constituent molecules available to other organisms. Bacteria in the roots of certain plants, such as peas and beans, fix nitrogen gas from the air into organic nitrogen, required by plants. Other bacteria live in the guts of herbivores, such as cows, helping them digest grass by breaking down its cellulose[a] cell walls. Within the human gut, there are billions of bacteria and other single-celled organisms. These help digest our food and can even produce vitamins. A typical person may contain more bacterial cells than human ones!

---

[a] Cellulose is an indigestible plant fibre made from the sugar glucose.

Bacterial cells generally do not need to cooperate with other cells: they are able to act for their own benefit. In this respect, we might describe them as 'selfish'. This is not a value judgement; it just means their task is to reproduce more of their own kind. Given the opportunity, a bacterial cell on your skin will form a colony. The result might be a pimple, or a rampant, flesh-eating infection. To bacteria, your body is just a place to grow and spread, as rapidly as conditions allow.

Cooperative cells

Unlike bacteria, the body of each human, or other animal or plant, contains billions of cells. We begin with just two: an ovum, or egg, from the mother, and a sperm from the father. These fuse to form a single cell that multiplies and develops into a baby, over the next nine months. Beneath the baby's skin is an incredible organisation of tissues, which is more complex than anything ever designed by people.

Scientists do not fully understand the process of forming a baby from a single fertilised egg. We do know, however, that it involves a controlled sequence of cellular change, growth and cell death. The egg divides many times and resulting cells respond to chemical signals, to change into muscle cells, nerve cells or bone cells, for example. Consider the biceps muscle, in the upper arm. Originally, all its cells are stem cells, which can turn into any type of tissue. Cells in the right location receive signals from other cells in the surrounding tissues, telling them to become muscle cells. For this to happen, the cells must recognise and obey the signals.

Some cells are signalled to grow and divide rapidly, while others are told to commit suicide, to help form the shape of the body. The end result is a structure of unimaginable intricacy. A single organ, such as the human brain, is more complex than the most powerful computer. This fantastic level of organisation is achieved through cells sending and receiving simple chemical signals, and agreeing to cooperate with each other.

Our cells' cooperative nature is not an accident, it is essential to our existence. In order to grow a body, human cells engage in carefully orchestrated agreement. Later, bodily maintenance involves the same processes of cell signalling, growth and cell death, as even the tiniest cut needs to be repaired. Small injuries can be fixed without a scar or any sign of damage. Repair of such wounds calls for detailed information about the structure of the tissue. There is no simple map to guide the cells: the result occurs because of cellular organisation and cooperation.

How did our cells gain the ability to work together in this way? Perhaps, hundreds of millions of years ago, groups of single cells started to cluster together. Grouping can offer advantages: birds flock to avoid predators, for example. Clumping could have helped those formerly single cells to survive and propagate. Such cooperation was a difficult transition for evolution to achieve. It could have taken in the region of two billion years for single-celled creatures to learn to work together as a simple organism.

To gain maximum advantage, cells that group together need to cooperate. A flock of birds stays together because each bird flies with the flock, rather than going off in a direction of its own. In a similar way, once a clump was advantageous to survival, stickier cells would be more likely to persist, whereas slippery cells would tend to drift away. In a sense, the stickier cell is cooperative and the slippery cell is more independent or selfish.

Over millions of years, the clumps of cells evolved into highly structured organisms. Such organisms can have clear advantages over single cells. For example, animals with legs can move to a more favourable environment. However, the increased cooperation necessary to create the structure may be disadvantageous to particular individual cells.

Some cells might be directed to commit suicide, sacrificing themselves for the good of the whole. If such a cell were able, it might refuse to cooperate, choosing instead to leave the clump. As multicellular plants and animals evolved, there has always have been the risk that any particular cell would become selfish. Each cell is pulled in two directions: towards cooperation or autonomy.

If the cells were genetically different, then there would be little advantage to a cell that agreed to sacrifice itself for the good of the whole. However, if the cells were all genetically identical offspring of a single cell, then altruistic behaviour might act to increase the survival of the shared genes. In this case, self-sacrifice would make that particular cell line more likely to survive.

Selfish cells

If large numbers of mutations occur in a clump of cells, the offspring become genetically different.[b] As genetic differences increase, cells

---

[b] A mutation is a change, resulting from error in, or damage to, a gene.

become more individual and less like the group from which they originated. When two cells are sufficiently different, they start to evolve separately and compete for survival.

Cancer cells are cells that have become selfish. They behave with many of the characteristics of single-celled organisms. Cancer cells do not respond to control signals: they grow in an unrestrained way and avoid committing suicide. Cancer is a form of abnormal cell growth. It is as if the cancer cell has become a new species of single-celled organism: a selfish cell. Such selfish cells compete with each other and with healthy tissue cells. In some rare cases, this competition may destroy the viability of the tumour producing a spontaneous regression. In most cases, the cells grow and invade other tissues and, left untreated, will ultimately destroy the host.

Cancer is a consequence of our evolution from single to multi-cellular beings. Any individual cell can break away from its growth controls and revert to an earlier, selfish form. Evolution dictates that if the genes in a particular cell differ greatly from those of the host, they will behave selfishly and may act in a way that we describe as cancer.

How cancer grows

'Nothing in this world is to be feared... only understood.' Marie Curie

Cancer cells are formed when cells divide with errors. Within the body, healthy cells multiply continuously. For example, stem cells in our skin, bone marrow, or intestines divide to form new tissue.

Cells with genetic errors, or that divide imperfectly, will produce abnormal offspring. If these produce further offspring, then more cells will carry the abnormality. As the process of erroneous cell division continues, the resulting offspring become more and more different from the original cells. Like a new species, these cells cease cooperating with the healthy tissues and increase their number uncontrollably; they have become selfish cells.

This conversion of healthy cells to selfish cells, or cancer, depends on the availability of antioxidants.

Antioxidants

Antioxidants are fashionable additions to foods and cosmetics. However, the recent interest in these substances is based on science. An antioxidant, as the name suggests, is something that prevents oxidation.

Oxidation is a chemical processes, which scientists originally thought involved combination of a substance with oxygen. For example, iron is oxidised to iron oxide (rust) by the addition of oxygen. Fire is an oxidation process and occurs when substances are heated in the presence of oxygen. Other examples include high explosives, such as dynamite, which gain their power from rapid oxidation reactions.

Oxidation was named after the gas oxygen, which was thought to be essential for such reactions. Although scientists now know that oxidation reactions can occur when no oxygen is present, we still use the historical term oxidation to describe particular kinds of chemical reactions.

Oxidation and its opposite, reduction, can also be explained in terms of loss or gain of subatomic particles, called electrons. Most people are familiar with electrons as the carriers of electricity. Oxidation occurs when a substance loses electrons, reduction when a substance gains electrons.[a] Oxidation and reduction occur together: when one substance loses electrons, another gains them. Such simultaneous processes are called redox (reduction-oxidation) reactions.

Biological oxidation processes are often less dramatic than those we learn about in chemistry. A classic example is the flesh of an apple turning brown (oxidising), when cut and exposed to air. Oxygen in the air reacts with the apple's surface, removing electrons. However, an antioxidant, such as vitamin C, can donate electrons to the apple, replacing those lost to the air. Thus, browning can be delayed by painting the surface with a vitamin C solution. In making a fruit salad, a cook might use lemon juice, which contains vitamin C, to keep the apples nice and white.

Antioxidants are often described as preventing free radical tissue damage. In the body, a *free radical* is a molecule that has lost an electron and needs to 'steal' another from elsewhere. When a free radical steals an electron from another molecule, it often creates another free radical, as the molecule that has lost its electron needs to steal one in turn. Such a chain of electron loss can end up oxidising an essential part of the cell's machinery, such as a gene's DNA,[b] or a protein.[c] However, antioxidants can prevent such damage by giving up an electron to a free radical, thus breaking the chain.

Free radicals

Free radicals damage tissues by stealing electrons, which causes oxidation. X-Rays, sunburn and some anticancer drugs generate free radicals in tissues. In general, tissue oxidation and free radical damage are not good things; many people take antioxidant supplements to prevent them.

Not all oxidants are bad - some are essential to life. People and other animals cannot live for more than a few minutes without a supply of oxygen to our tissues. This is used to oxidise our food, generating energy and producing electrons for antioxidants. White blood cells also generate useful oxidants, releasing them to protect us against bacteria and viruses.[d]

---

[a] Mnemonic: OIL RIG – Oxidation Is Loss, Reduction Is Gain (of electrons).
[b] Genes are long sequences of DNA, which stands for deoxyribonucleic acid. A gene contains the information for building a protein.
[c] Proteins are the main "toolkit" of the cell and are used to provide structure or, as enzymes, to help chemical reactions.
[d] A virus is a small particle, made of genes and protein, which can infect a cell.

These white blood cells contain higher levels of antioxidants, such as vitamin C, than most other cells. They need the extra antioxidants to protect themselves from the oxidants and free radicals they produce to kill germs.

High levels of oxidants, even those produced by our own immune systems, can be damaging. The red and swollen nose that accompanies a cold is an example of inflammation caused by oxidation. Our immune system fights the invading virus, but the infection and the body's response generate free radicals, inflammation and discomfort.

Not all free radicals and oxidants produced in our tissues are damaging, however. Our cells use low concentrations of several oxidants and free radicals to signal to each other. For example, a minute amount of an oxidant, such as hydrogen peroxide, may be used to tell nearby cells to divide more rapidly.

Cell growth

In order to maintain a stable tissue structure, cells need to grow and divide. The control of cell growth has evolved over millions of years. The body's cells are bombarded with *grow* and *don't grow* signals, though most are maintained in a relatively stable state by signals not to grow.

Numerous genes make sure that control of cell growth and division is finely tuned. Some genes have been found to promote cancer; these, known as oncogenes, become active when growth is needed. Cancer cells that express these particular genes have a growth advantage.[e]

Other genes slow down or inhibit cell growth; these are called tumour suppressor genes. Healthy cells typically express tumour suppressor genes, ensuring they do not grow or divide unless it is essential. Cancer cells often lose or inhibit these suppressor genes, which then do not prevent or slow the growth of the tumour.

Redox control

Experiments with cell cultures have helped scientists understand the processes of cell growth. A cell culture is a population of cells in a solution, or on a dish of nutrient jelly. If a low concentration of an

----

[e] Cells contain many genes, units of hereditary information, not all of which are active. Cells that 'express' particular genes are those that show the characteristics associated with those genes.

oxidant, such as hydrogen peroxide, is applied to a culture of human cells, they divide more frequently. Low levels of oxidants are typically signals for the cell to divide. Similarly, antioxidants, such as vitamin C, often inhibit or slow cell growth and division.[f]

These *grow* and *stop growing* signals are converted to similar redox signals inside the cell. Within the cell, there are various compartments, such as the cell nucleus. Each compartment can have its own redox state. These intracellular redox states help control whether the cell will divide. In general, raised levels of oxidation promote cell division, whereas a reducing state, high in antioxidants, inhibits cell division.

Cell death

Cells can be signalled, or requested, to commit suicide. Since dying is the last thing a cell does, signals for cell death need to be clear and unambiguous. It would not be good for health if cells were dying unnecessarily. On receiving signals to commit suicide, the cell must evaluate them and only act if it is sure the message is valid. If the cell determines that the message is correct, it starts a program of cell death, called apoptosis.

We have already described how cell death by apoptosis is an essential part of the development of our bodily structures. Apoptosis has another, vitally important, role: the prevention of cancer. If a cell is dividing too rapidly, it can be signalled to commit suicide. Even more strangely, a cell that is dividing too rapidly can elect to bring about its own death.

We have seen that as the oxidation state of the cell rises, cell division increases. Rapidly dividing cells have increased levels of oxidants, such as hydrogen peroxide, which are essential to cell division. However, if a cell becomes abnormal and is dividing too quickly, its oxidation state increases still further, acting as a signal for the cell to kill itself.

To recap, in healthy cells, raised levels of oxidation can initiate cell division, but even higher levels signal the start of apoptosis. If a cancer is to flourish, therefore, it needs to inhibit or disable the cell suicide mechanism.

---

[f] Thus, antioxidants might delay the development of cancer cells.

The balance of growth

A tumour forms when abnormal cells increase in number and form a lump. This can happen when the cells divide more rapidly than normal, or if they die less often. Both cell division and cell death are controlled, at least in part, by the balance of oxidants and antioxidants. This observation leads to an understanding of how cancer may be treated.

Although cancer is an abnormal growth of tissue, it remains subject to the basic laws of biology. The most important idea in biology is evolution. So, before we consider the possibility of curing the disease, we need to examine the evolutionary pressures on the growth of a population of abnormal cells in the body.

Cancer is the abnormal growth of abnormal cells. This growth can occur because the abnormal cells divide more rapidly and they refuse to die. Antioxidants can prevent cancer by inhibiting cell division. Inflammation and tissue damage produce oxidation and cell proliferation. Local oxidants, like hydrogen peroxide, can kill cancer cells.

The evolution of cancer

'When you hear hoofbeats in Texas,
think horses not zebras' Anonymous

Cancer cells act for their own survival, rather than that of their host. We can think of these selfish cancer cells as a new species, growing autonomously in the environment of the body.

Evolution acts on every animal and plant. Evolutionary selection pressure applies both to the individual organism and its component parts. Thus, cells in our bodies are subject to selection pressure, since they can grow and divide as individuals. As long as cells respond to *grow/stop-growing* signals, they remain under the body's control. But if a cell starts dividing to produce a tumour, evolution comes into play. Cells with different genetic expression, growth and behaviour compete against other cells, including those of the host body.

Damage and errors

Injury to a tissue can damage its cells. Sometimes this damage is genetic and affects the DNA of the cell. When this happens, the errors or mutations are passed on to the cell's offspring.

A classical approach to cancer considers the minimum number of mutations required to produce a cancer cell. Scientists have estimated that this minimum might be five or six. However, this approach often assumes that such mutations damage the cell's error correction mechanisms, leading to a cascade of damage in descendant cells. In other words, the model does not mean that cancer cells differ from normal cells by only a few mutations, but that the five or six mutations generate many more during the division process. The initial mutations lead to a cascade of further mutation in the cell's descendants. Each generation of cells has more genetic damage.

Damage to the mechanisms of cell division can also cause problems, which are passed on to daughter cells. For example, cells' genetic material, DNA, is contained in tiny objects called chromosomes.[a] When a human cell divides, its 23 chromosomes are duplicated; one complete set then passes to each of the daughter cells. However, if the division process

---

[a] Human cells contain 46 duplicate chromosomes in 23 pairs.

is damaged, an unequal number of chromosomes can be passed to the daughter cells.[b] In the extreme condition, two copies (46 chromosome pairs) could be passed to one daughter cell and none to the other. Chromosomes may also be broken, in which case fragments of chromosomes could be inherited.

Chromosome damage is common in cancer cells and appears universal in malignant tumours. Malignant tumours spread rapidly and are more dangerous. Typically, cancer cells have massive genetic changes, along with abnormal numbers of chromosomes. This is interesting, because variation in the chromosome number is one of the few ways a new species can be produced quickly.

Botanists think that half of all flowering plant species arose as a result of chromosome duplication. If an organism has big changes to its DNA, its properties differ from those of the original, sufficiently for it to be described as a new species. This analogy is an informative way of thinking about cancer. A cancer is something like an infective organism that is derived from our own cells.

Proliferation

In our discussion of the cell damage involved in causing cancer, we assumed the cell would be dividing. Cell division is central to models of cancer generation. Cancer, after all, is defined as abnormal cellular growth. However, another factor is equally essential to producing cancer. This is a mechanism to generate errors and damage inside the cell. Following this, cell division must propagate and increase the damage throughout the offspring.

The theory of evolution describes how mutations can accumulate through passing generations. This is often described as 'survival of the fittest.' Evolution relates to competition between organisms, over generations. An organism that leaves more offspring, which can reproduce successfully, is more fit. In this context, the word 'fit' means able to survive and breed.[c]

---

[b] A well-known example is Down's Syndrome. During division, one sperm or egg accidentally gets both copies of chromosome 21, while the other daughter cell gets none. If the cell with both combines with a normal cell, the result is three – a condition known as trisomy 21, which causes Down's syndrome.

[c] Surprisingly, the slang expression 'he (or she) is fit', meaning sexually attractive or 'hot', is quite close to Darwin's meaning, although Darwin also included the idea of being well adapted to a particular environment.

Natural selection favours organisms based on their ability to leave offspring and make best use of available resources. The same is required for a cancer cell to become malignant. By definition, cancer cells leave more offspring than healthy cells. They use up available resources to fuel their growth, until they destroy their environment which, in this case, is the patient.

Although we are talking about evolution, we are not concerned with the origins of life or how organisms have developed over millions of years. Rather, we are interested in rapid changes in cells, to produce something like a new species, in a short period of time. The changes required for a cell to become cancerous are those needed for the evolutionary success of any single-celled organism, namely, increased growth and proliferation. Once the processes of increased cell division and inherited errors are combined, evolution takes over, favouring just those cells with the characteristics of malignant cancer.

Benign growth

At first, erroneous cell division produces a distinct tissue mass, called a benign tumour. Benign tumours are relatively safe; they grow locally and do not invade distant parts of the body. Benign tumours may grow slowly, to a limited size. Often, they remain subject to the body's controls, not to grow too large or too quickly. Despite this, benign tumours can occasionally threaten the host's well-being, by growing excessively large or by interfering with the function of affected organs.[d]

Cells in benign tumours are generally similar to the original cells from which they formed. Benign tumour cells have not become sufficiently different from healthy cells, either genetically or behaviourally, to be classified as a new species. Such cells differ from normal cells but remain cooperative with cellular controls. Benign cells are assertive, rather than selfish.

Malignant growth

By contrast, malignant cancer cells show signs of massive change, and it is often difficult to tell from which type of cell they originated. A typical malignant tumour contains populations of widely differing cells. Even features such as the number of chromosomes, which are usually

---

[d] An example of a benign tumour causing harm is small tumours in the womb, called uterine fibroids, that may lead to excessive menstrual blood loss and consequent anaemia.

characteristic of the species, can vary widely. Within the same tumour, cancer cells may range from having only half the normal number of chromosomes to having multiple sets. These cells compete with each other, as well as with the host. The cell that is able to grow quickly and leave most offspring is the winner – in the short term!

A growing malignant cancer is like an ecosystem of organisms, each competing for survival. A successful cell leaves more offspring. Those that can spread and colonise other parts of the body have a particular advantage. Malignancy is the term we use to describe the result of successful evolutionary competition, leading to a population of selfish cells.

Cancer grows by a process of microevolution, which depends on cells dividing with errors. Factors that increase cell proliferation increase the risk of developing cancer, as does any insult or damage to the cells. Factors such as X-Rays, which can damage the genes or cell division controls, are particularly dangerous. Benign tumours contain cells that are similar to healthy cells and grow into a relatively safe, local, lump. Malignant cells differ from healthy cells both genetically and in their structure. They are particularly invasive and dangerous to the host.

Nutrition and prevention

'God heals and the doctor takes the fees.' Benjamin Franklin

Cancer is largely a disease of ageing. As we get older, the chance of developing cancer increases rapidly. Indeed, age is probably the greatest risk factor for the development of cancer.

Nutrition offers approaches to both prevention and treatment. However, these two are quite different. For prevention, the aim is to provide optimal nutrition for the patient. By contrast, nutritional therapy aims to control or destroy cancer cells, while making sure that nutrition intended for the patient does not provide the cancer with the nutrients it needs to grow.

Some scientists have suggested that what we eat is a bigger risk factor for cancer than smoking. People are generally aware that avoiding smoking and other established risk factors will help them avoid cancer. However, it is estimated that 30-40% of all cancers have a dietary origin. For this reason, people wanting to lower their risk of getting cancer, or those who have a predisposition to the disease, may choose to modify their diet. For such people, consumption of a range of antioxidants, from both food and dietary supplements, is the first step.

Although we present a summary of vitamins and other nutrients that might help prevent cancer, we are not suggesting that anyone should take all those on the list. Neither is this a complete and authoritative list of supplements; rather, it is a guide. Essentially, the aim in prevention is for the person to be well nourished, with a high intake of a range of antioxidants.

Nutrient deficiency

Deficiencies in the diet can greatly increase the chances of developing cancer. This is particularly the case for antioxidant vitamins and minerals. Some individual nutrients, such as vitamin D_3, which is created by the action of sunlight on the skin, have a particular role to play in prevention. Although exposure to sunlight can lead to skin cancer, people who avoid the sun completely might increase their risk of other forms of cancer, through lack of vitamin D_3. Recent advice to stay out of the sun may have been premature and, unless people are supplementing with vitamin D_3, could increase overall cancer rates.

Standard advice to eat less and ensure that the diet is varied, with a high intake of vegetables, is to be encouraged. In addition, dietary supplementation with relatively high levels of vitamins and minerals is likely to be beneficial. However, the quality and amount of substances in commercially available supplements is variable. The cost of a high quality, 'natural' multi-vitamin and multi-mineral tablet is well spent. Often, supermarket multivitamins are low quality formulations that may not be absorbed well and may contain other, potentially damaging, chemicals such as artificial sweeteners. For example, some low-cost multivitamin tablets contain government recommended minimum amounts (RDA)[a] levels of vitamin E. Often, this vitamin E is synthetic and is less effective than mixed, natural forms, which are also available.

Some authorities have advised against the use of supplements. Such advice does not take into account the risks associated with even marginal deficiency. Deficiency of any one of the following causes DNA damage: folic acid, vitamin B6, Vitamin B12, vitamin B3 (niacin), vitamin C, vitamin E, iron or zinc. This damage is significant and its effects are similar to those of ionising radiation.[b] Such malnutrition is likely to be a major cause of cancer. At the back of this book we recommend some books on optimal nutrition. However, nutritionists or even suitably qualified staff at your local health food outlet could provide guidance.

---

[a] RDA officially stands for Recommended Dietary Allowance but is often referred to as Ridiculous Dietary Allowance by more informed nutritionists.
[b] Ames B.N. (2001) DNA damage from micronutrient deficiencies is likely to be a major cause of cancer, Mutat Res, 475(1-2), 7-20.

Multivitamins

	Formulation	Approximate Dose
Vitamin A	Retinyl palmitate	10,000 iu
Vitamin B1	Thiamine	100 mg
Vitamin B2	Riboflavin	100 mg
Vitamin B3	Niacinamide	100 mg
Vitamin B5	Pantothenic acid	50 mg
Vitamin B6	Pyridoxine hydrochloride	50 mg
Vitamin B7 / H	Biotin	80 µg
Vitamin B9	Folic acid	400 µg
Vitamin B12	Cyanocobalamin	100 µg
Vitamin D	Cholecalciferol	400 iu
Vitamin K	Phylloquinone (K1) or menaquinone (K2)	90 µg
PABA	Para-aminobenzoic acid	80 mg

This table is intended as a guide to the range and doses of nutrients that a multivitamin tablet might contain. Vitamin K is contraindicated in people who are taking anticoagulants (blood thinners, such as warfarin), breast feeding or pregnant. Similarly, pregnant women should not take high dose vitamin A supplements, such as those indicated in this table. Multivitamins often contain poor quality vitamin E; for this reason we have not listed vitamin E in this table.

Multi-minerals

	Formulation	Approximate Dose
Chromium	Chromium polynicotinate	100 µg
Iodine	Potassium iodide	150 µg
Magnesium	Magnesium citrate	350 mg
Manganese	Manganese chelate	2 mg
Molybdenum	Sodium molybdate	35 µg
Selenium	Methylselenocysteine	200 µg
Zinc	Zinc chelate	25 mg

This table gives suggestions for what forms of minerals and additional supplements might be considered.

Note that we have not included copper or iron. Iron supplements may be useful in pregnancy or in the treatment of anaemia but are not recommended as a general supplement. Copper, although essential, can be a source of oxidation and is therefore not included in this table. Both iron and copper supplements may be useful in cancer treatment, however.

Phytonutrients

	Substance	Example source
Carotenoids	alpha-carotene, beta-carotene, beta-cryptoxanthin, lycopene, lutein, zeaxanthin	Carrots, tomatoes
Chlorophyll		Green plants
Chlorophyllin		
Organosulphates	gamma-glutamylcysteines, cysteine sulfoxides	Garlic and onion
Flavonoids	cyanidin, delphinidin, malvidin, pelargonidin, peonidin, petunidin, proanthocyanidins	Chocolate, tea, grapes, red wine
Flavanols	catechin, epicatechin gallate, epigallocatechin gallate, theaflavins, thearubigins	Black, green and white teas
Flavanones	hesperetin, naringenin, eriodictyol	Citrus fruit
Flavonols	isorhamnetin, kaempferol, myricetin, quercetin,	Onions, broccoli and teas
Flavones	apigenin, luteolin	Herbs and spices

Carbohydrates

Cancer cells are preferentially nourished by glucose, as opposed to other nutrients. Since the body breaks down sugars and starches to form glucose, consumption of these foods helps to feed developing cancer cells. Thus, one way to reduce the risk of cancer formation is to eat less sugars and carbohydrates. This can be difficult, as such foods are addictive.

Most people think of sugar as the substance we add to tea or coffee. Such intakes can be reduced in stages: for example, a person who currently takes two spoonfuls might lower the amount by half a spoonful a week. However, this is only the tip of the iceberg; many of our favourite foods contain carbohydrates. The widespread use of sweet and starchy substances in convenience foods makes it hard to cut down on these.

Carbohydrates include starches, which are found in pasta, potatoes, bread, cereals and many western foods. Perhaps more surprisingly, sugars such as fructose, which is found in fruit, and lactose, contained in milk, are also carbohydrates. Cutting down on these sources involves switching to a low carbohydrate diet. This might consist of meat, poultry, fish, eggs, oils, butter, non-starchy salads, green vegetables, avocado pears, certain nuts and seeds. Since fats are not excluded (within reason), such a diet is not unpalatable. Low carbohydrate diets are popular, so it should not be hard to find one that suits you.

If you can't live without your carbs, choose foods which release them slowly, such as those with a low glycaemic index (low GI). Eat small quantities of citrus fruit, apple, apricot, cherry, peach, pear, plum, berries or kiwi, rather than sweet fruits such as banana, peach, grapes, melon, mango or pineapple. Eat fruit whole, rather than drinking it as juice, which has a higher GI. Again, there are many books which will tell you how to select low GI foods.

Antioxidants

Since cell division can be stimulated by oxidants and inhibited by antioxidants, an antioxidant-rich diet lowers the risk of developing cancer. Such a diet includes a variety of fruit and vegetables, and a simple rule is to choose those with a range of strong colours. The colours in foods such as broccoli, red cabbage, raspberries, blueberries, tomatoes, and green tea indicate the presence of antioxidants, called phytonutrients. Carotenoids, for example, are yellow, orange and red pigments, synthesized by plants. Perhaps the best known of these is beta-carotene, found in carrots.

Even for those who consume adequate amounts of fresh fruit and vegetables, dietary supplementation may be helpful. In particular, a high intake of vitamin C supports the action of other dietary antioxidants. Many of these, including beta-carotene, can donate an electron to prevent tissue oxidation, but then cease to act as antioxidants until they replace their lost electron. High doses of vitamin C provide a 'free' source of electrons, which can recharge other antioxidants. Vitamin C is the primary factor in antioxidant nutrition.

We have recently shown that many of the myths surrounding high dose vitamin C are false. These include suggestions that high doses cause kidney stones, do not prevent colds, or merely create "expensive urine" by wastefully excreting vitamin C.[c] In fact, scientific evidence is consistent with the optimal intake for a typical, healthy, young adult being at least 2-3 grams per day, taken in divided doses. This may be achieved by taking 500-1000mg, with each meal, or at tea or coffee breaks. However, some people may require more: up to about 20 grams per day. The aim is to set up a dynamic flow of vitamin C, delivering antioxidant electrons to the body. A person's nutritional requirements, genetics and biochemistry are to some extent specific to the individual.

The table of phytonutrients gives a small indication of the vast number of plant chemicals that could play a part in the prevention and treatment of cancer. Unfortunately, research into the medicinal properties of these substances is limited. However, what results are available indicate that large numbers of safe anticancer agents are contained in plants. An example is curcumin, found in the spice turmeric, which gives curries their yellow colour. Turmeric has been used medicinally in India for hundreds of years but, in the west, interest in its therapeutic properties is recent.

Healthy people, or those with increased risk of cancer, can help themselves by eating a balanced diet. The diet should be low in carbohydrates and contain a range of vegetables. Supplementing with a high quality multivitamin formula and with antioxidants is easy to achieve, with minimal changes in lifestyle. In particular, a dynamic flow of vitamin C will help drive the body into a healthy, reduced state.

[c] Hickey S. Roberts H. (2004) Ascorbate: The Science of Vitamin C, Lulu Press.

Putting tumours on a diet

'The practice of physic is jostled by quacks on the one side, and by science on the other.' Edward Abbey

Many doctors believe that changes in diet have little effect on the life expectancy of cancer patients. This medical myth was expressed recently by Jonathan Waxman, Professor of Oncology at Imperial College, London:

'... once cancer has been diagnosed no change in diet will lead to any improvement in cancer outcomes. In a recent review of 59 randomised trials of dietary manoeuvres in cancer no evidence was found that supported this approach.' [a]

Waxman's unscientific claim that 'no change in diet will lead to any improvement in cancer outcomes' is not supported by the evidence he cites.[b] Indeed, unless he tested every possible dietary change, Waxman could not support this assertion! The cited review's authors conclude that 'the impact of most nutritional interventions cannot be reliably estimated, because of the limited number of trials, many of which were of low quality.' They add that 'there is no evidence that dietary modification by cancer patients improves survival and benefits disease prognosis.'

We should stress that 'no evidence' means just that – there is no evidence, one way or the other. Waxman's extrapolation from the reviewers' position of 'no evidence' to his claim that 'no change in diet will lead to improvements' is unsubstantiated. In fact, the medical community has not properly tested appropriate nutritional therapies in cancer patients.

Don't feed the cancer

Although we do not agree with Professor Waxman's sweeping generalisation, there is certainly misinformation in the field of nutrition

---

[a] Waxman J. (2006) Shark Cartilage in the Water, BMJ, 333, 1129.
[b] Waxman did not give the reference, which is: Davies A. *et al* (2006) Nutritional interventions and outcome in patients with cancer or preinvasive lesions: systematic review, J Natl Cancer Inst, 98(14), 961-973.

and cancer. Most books, including those from reputable sources, urge cancer patients to ensure they have excellent nutrition, on the grounds that a well-nourished body will be better able to ward off the disease. Other authors suggest that nutrients to boost the immune system will be of particular benefit. This sounds like common sense, but is not necessarily the best way to combat cancer.

To understand this, we need to realise that tumours contain a range of cells. Some are actively dividing; some appear to be doing nothing, while others are dying. However, for a cancer to grow, more cells must be created than die.

Growing tissues, including cancer cells, require nutrients. A dividing cell needs the energy and materials to create a copy of itself. If insufficient resources are available, cell division will be delayed. Thus, depriving cancer cells of nutrients may inhibit cell division and also increase cell deaths.

Conversely, food consumed by patients may help feed the cancer, because cancer cells are derived from ordinary body cells; both require nutrients to grow. All cells, whether they are malignant or healthy, need glucose, proteins, vitamins and minerals. To reduce the risk that nutrients may benefit the cancer preferentially, cancer patients should not consume an excess of any substance which helps cancers to grow.

Since cancer cells need food, the question arises whether we could starve a cancer to death? Clearly, such an approach would not be sensible if the patient also starved. Fortunately, there are differences in the nutritional requirements of tumours, compared to healthy tissue.

Fast-growing tumours have similarities to children: both are particularly susceptible to the effects of starvation. If children are deprived of nutrients during sensitive growth-spurt periods, their growth can be stunted permanently. Under starvation conditions, adults last longer. In the same way, a growing tumour may be more vulnerable to malnutrition than its adult host. We can use this information to benefit the patient, at the expense of the cancer.

Raw vegetables inhibit cancer?

In the late 1970's, when Dr Arthur Robinson was President of the Linus Pauling Institute, he performed a set of experiments on mice with cancer. His aim was to test claims that a diet of raw vegetables could slow cancer growth, helping patients survive longer. Although the scientists did not think this was possible, their job was to consider and test the ideas, with open minds.

The results were surprising: mice on a diet of raw vegetables developed fewer and less severe tumours than control mice on a regular diet. Addition of protein-rich nuts and seeds to the experimental diet reduced the anticancer effect. Paradoxically, the likely reason for these findings was not that vegetables provide better nutrition but, rather, that raw vegetables are hard to digest. The experimental mice were deficient in nutrients: their diet was so poor that the cancers were unable to grow.

Cancers need sugar

Cancer cells differ from healthy cells in several consistent ways. For a start, cancer cells tend to be anaerobic, which means they use less oxygen and burn more sugar than healthy cells.[c]

By contrast, typical human cells are aerobic: they need oxygen from the air to survive. This oxygen is used to metabolise (burn) food, producing energy. Perhaps surprisingly, high levels of oxygen are poisonous, so our cells contain a range of antioxidants, to protect them from oxidation.

Being anaerobic, cancer cells are less dependent on oxygen to burn food. Cancer cells use a simpler, but less efficient, form of metabolism; they depend preferentially on glucose for energy, whereas healthy cells use a variety of food sources. Cancer cells also have relatively poor antioxidant defences, so they are less able to protect themselves from oxygen damage.

In the experiment described above, a diet of raw vegetables and fruit starved the mice of nutrients, providing only small amounts of sugar and protein. Under these conditions, the tumours were unable to grow. Although the reduced quantities of sugar and other nutrients did not destroy the tumours, they remained small.

Such results are not unique. In another experiment, researchers gave mice with cancer different amounts of sugar and waited 70 days, to see how many would survive.[d] Of the mice with high blood sugar, only 8 out of 24 (33%) survived. Those with normal blood sugar levels were more

---

[c] There are two types of animal cells: anaerobic and aerobic. Aerobic cells need oxygen, whereas oxygen is poisonous to anaerobic cells. This is a basic classification for life on earth.
[d] Santisteban G.A. et al (1985) Glycemic modulation of tumor tolerance in a mouse model of breast cancer, Biochem Biophys Res Commun, 132(3), 1174-1179.

fortunate: 16 out of 24 (67%) survived. By contrast, almost all the mice with low blood sugar survived: 19 out of 20 (95%).

If similar results could be demonstrated in humans, then lowering carbohydrate intake would give cancer patients a far greater life expectancy than current treatments, such as chemotherapy.

Starvation

The surgeon who brought the raw vegetable diet to the attention of Pauling and Robinson learnt about it from one of his own patients. This patient took the diet to the limit: his doctor described him as looking like a concentration camp victim. However, after months of food restriction, the cancer had disappeared and the patient was alive, against the odds. The doctor helped his patient regain weight, and the cancer did not return.

Since this example is extreme, we must stress that starvation can kill. Long term dietary restriction is a serious matter, not to be confused with a simple weight loss diet. Currently, we do not know how much dietary restriction might be necessary to prevent the growth of a typical tumour. It could be that restricting carbohydrate and calorie intake would be almost as effective as a raw vegetable diet. It is also possible that restricting specific nutrients, such as iron, would be effective; there is some evidence for this. Further research, including clinical trials, is essential.

Patients considering dietary restriction as an approach to cancer have several options. They could limit their intake of carbohydrates and calories. They could refuse nutritional supplements, except for those known to inhibit cancer growth. They could replace parts of their diet with raw vegetables. Ultimately, they could elect to live on a diet composed entirely of raw vegetables, with high levels of specific anticancer supplements, such as selenium or vitamin C.

Contrary to many books on nutrition, we caution against the use of juices. Authors who believed the benefits of their diets were attributable to a property known as 'goodness' in fruits and vegetables, decided to make it easier for patients, by recommending juicing the vegetables. Unfortunately, from a cancer treatment viewpoint, this increases the availability of nutrients and carbohydrates. If you eat a raw apple, its nutrients are released slowly in the gut. Apple cells have strong walls, protecting their contents from digestion. Juicing breaks down the cell walls, so apple juice tastes sweet and is full of nutrients. It is great for healthy people wanting to avoid cancer, but totally unsuitable as a nutrient-deficient component of a cancer treatment plan.

Whatever level of approach they undertake, patients would be wise to ask a physician, or other suitably qualified health practitioner, to monitor their progress carefully.

Optimal nutrition for a cancer patient may be quite different to that of a healthy person. It is possible to slow cancer growth by restricting nutrients in the diet. With the correct diet, a cancer can be starved, while the patient remains reasonably well-nourished. This does not mean cancer patients should starve themselves to further ill health. A diet of raw vegetables appears to be effective against cancer growth; a similar effect might be achieved by restricting sugar, iron or specific nutrients.

Controlling cancer

'We can endure neither our evils nor their cures.' Livy

The aim of cancer treatment is to extend the life of the patient, while controlling disease symptoms. Ideally, the quality of life should be high, so the therapy should not cause the patient to suffer debilitating side effects.

The science of biology suggests two ways for people to survive cancer, while maintaining a good quality of life. The first is to eliminate the population of cancer cells. In biological terms, this means driving the cancer to extinction, so no cells remain in the body. The second is to stop the cancer growing, so the person's life continues, relatively unaffected. This second approach, which involves living with the cancer, can effectively turn a malignant cancer into a comparatively harmless tumour.

Surgery

As a treatment, surgery has one great advantage over radiation and chemotherapy: it removes the cancer from the body. If the cancer is caught early and has not spread, surgery can stop the disease. Surgeons cure early cancers by removing the tumour and some surrounding tissue. However, when the disease has spread, or metastasised, to other parts of the body, surgery will typically not provide a cure. Although major growths can be removed, other cancer cells, which have been left behind, can continue to grow.

In the majority of adult tumours, such as lung cancer, neither chemotherapy nor radiation-based treatments are commonly able to cure the disease. However, radiation and chemotherapy are often used in combination with surgery, in the hope of killing any residual cancerous cells.

Radiation

Radiation can be used in cases where surgery is not possible, as it can be applied to a larger area than surgery. High dose radiation kills cancer cells in a similar way to the redox therapy described in this book: both generate free radicals and oxidise the tumour.

Radiation creates damaging free radicals. Since cancer cells are slightly more sensitive to radiation than healthy tissues, they are less able to defend themselves against oxidation and free radical damage. When radiologists send beams of high energy X-rays or gamma rays through the affected area, these kill cancer cells preferentially. Unfortunately, some cancer cells are more resistant to radiation than others, and these cells can survive.

To destroy cancer, treatment needs to affect every cancer cell. Regrettably, cells which survive radiotherapy are often resistant to other therapies, including anticancer drugs. Like bacteria, which develop resistance to antibiotics, cancer treatment can result in cells which are multiply resistant to several forms of treatment.

Since X-rays can damage healthy tissues, doctors are not generally able to increase the dose of radiation until all cancer cells are destroyed. Some cancer cells survive at higher doses than can be tolerated by the patient. For this reason, the effectiveness of radiation is limited by its toxicity.

Chemotherapy

In theory, drugs for killing cancer have many advantages. Drugs are distributed throughout the body, so they can attack cancer cells in most tissues. Hence, while surgery is limited to removal of local tumours, drugs might be able to kill widespread cancers. In practice, conventional anticancer drugs kill healthy cells at doses not much greater than those which kill cancer. This means that the effectiveness of chemotherapy is limited by its toxicity.

Chemotherapeutic drugs often work by generating free radicals in the cancer cells. However, it is rare that drugs have only one action. Anticancer drugs can operate in additional ways, which poison or adversely affect healthy cells, leading to side effects. These limit the dose levels and the duration of therapy to those the patient can tolerate. Chemotherapy is generally not curative for solid tumours in adults. It is often used with surgery, in an attempt to kill remaining cells, after a tumour has been removed.

Both chemotherapy and radiation have practical limits. Such treatments kill susceptible cells, while leaving resistant cells unharmed. This process is similar to giving antibiotics for bacterial infections: if some bacteria survive, a drug-resistant infection can develop. Chemotherapy and radiation treatments tend to be given intermittently. In between cycles of therapy, or when the treatment is completed, resistant cells can multiply or stabilise. As a result, cycles of treatment become progressively less effective.

There is a popular myth that non-toxic anticancer agents are unavailable. In fact, they are common, easy to find and straightforward to study. We are at a loss to explain why non-toxic therapies are not a central part of cancer medicine.

Controlling cancer cells

As we have seen, it can be hard to drive a population of cancer cells to extinction without damaging the patient. Biologists study similar problems in animal populations. When rats are introduced to tropical islands, they sometimes out-compete indigenous species, eating the eggs of ground-nesting birds, for example. Once established, new species, such as rats, can be difficult to eradicate without harming the other animals on the island.

Even when pest control measures have apparently eliminated the rats, they can return. It may be possible to kill most of them but they breed rapidly. Even when no rats can be found, a few might remain, hidden from view. Yet as soon as conditions are favourable, the rat population can rebound rapidly. This pattern can be compared to a treatment that shrinks a tumour to undetectable levels, but does not stop it from recurring.

In such cases, we do not need to give up hope. Biologists have found that, even if it is impossible to remove all rats from an island, the numbers may be controlled. If there is a way to lower the number of rats sufficiently, other species can thrive. This is called population control. In a similar way, if we could control the growth of tumours, the patient might enjoy a prolonged, high quality life. In the long term, preventing tumour growth, without harming the patient, could make cancer a manageable disease.

Eradication of all cancer cells represents the extreme limit of cell population control. Halting or slowing growth, while less dramatic, could allow patients to survive for longer than they would otherwise have done. If a therapy that prevents cancer growth is not toxic to healthy cells, then it can be continued indefinitely. The patient may carry small tumours, but they might not be sufficient to threaten life or present symptoms.

There are two approaches to treating cancer. The first is to eradicate all malignant cells, providing a cure by driving the cancer to extinction. The second is population control. Such treatments encourage cancer cells to die, or inhibit cell growth and division. Tumours remain small enough not to affect health. In many cases, effective population control could provide an equivalent benefit to extinction, by extending life.

Vitamin C and cancer

'The philosophies of one age have become the absurdities of the next, and the foolishness of yesterday has become the wisdom of tomorrow.'
Sir William Osler

The role of vitamin C in cancer has been controversial for many years. However, in scientific terms, the controversy has largely been resolved. Substantial evidence shows that, in high enough doses, vitamin C will kill cancer cells while leaving healthy cells unharmed. This means vitamin C can form the basis of a non-toxic form of chemotherapy.

Many people are sceptical when they hear of vitamin C as a treatment for cancer. We agree - a gram or two per day will have little, if any, effect. In this context, we are talking about massive, pharmacological doses: up to 200g per day. Often, when we explain these levels, the scepticism is transferred from its possible effectiveness to the size of the dose.

An ideal anticancer drug

Ideally, an anticancer drug should have little or no toxicity. The dose could be increased to a level where it would kill cancer cells without harming the body. Such a drug would slow tumour growth or, gradually, kill the cancer cells. The patient could expect an extended life, with few side effects from the treatment.

A second feature of this imaginary anticancer drug might be its low price. Cancer therapy is notoriously expensive. An easily obtainable, inexpensive drug, not subject to drug company patents, would benefit patients.

Finally, our ideal anticancer treatment would be taken orally. Taking medicine in the form of a few pills or a refreshing drink has many advantages. Such a drug would need minimal direct clinical involvement. Patients would feel more in control of their therapy and of the disease. Obviously, the patient would need to be carefully monitored by competent physicians, with the advantages of modern diagnostic imaging and other techniques.

Not too long ago, this holy grail of chemotherapy seemed impossibly far away. Surprisingly, it may already exist.

In 1969, a scientist called Dean Burk found that high concentrations of vitamin C could kill cancer cells. He described vitamin C as potentially providing the beginnings of a new, non-toxic approach to chemotherapy. By the end of the 1960s, it was clear that the ideal anticancer drug was possible. Since that time, these results have been confirmed many times. The statement that vitamin C kills cancer cells, without harming normal cells, is no longer controversial.

Intravenous ascorbate

Scientists have shown, without doubt, that high concentrations of vitamin C can destroy cancer cells. When vitamin C is given intravenously, as sodium ascorbate, high blood levels can be achieved: high enough to kill most cancer cells. It has not yet been fully established that intravenous vitamin C extends the lives of cancer patients, but there is substantial evidence that it could.

Clearly, intravenous therapy must be carried out by a suitably qualified physician. Intravenous sodium ascorbate is a relatively safe alternative to conventional chemotherapy. An intravenous drip, containing, say, 75 grams of sodium ascorbate, might be given three times a week, over a five week cycle of therapy. Such a protocol is reported to shrink back many tumours, often to undetectable levels. When given appropriately, this therapy offers little risk of side effects - certainly less than those associated with conventional chemotherapy.

The main drawback of intravenous ascorbate is that delivery is intermittent. Unless the patient is in hospital, it may be impractical to give a continuous infusion of sodium ascorbate over a prolonged period of time. Usually, infusions lasting several hours are given for a period of a few weeks, in a cycle of treatment. A limitation of this approach is that, like conventional chemotherapy, it might shrink the tumour while selecting for resistant cells. If this happened, the stronger cells could re-grow once the treatment was over.

Intravenous treatment of cancer with sodium ascorbate should, therefore, be combined with dynamic flow level oral doses, to provide continuous selection pressure on the tumour.[a]

---

[a] Dynamic flow is achieved by taking frequent doses of vitamin C, to maintain high blood levels. Excess vitamin C flows through the body and is excreted in the urine. The actual dose varies from person to person, and depends on the state of health.

Oral doses

Oral doses of vitamin C may extend the life of cancer patients. However, vitamin C on its own is a relatively weak anticancer agent. A person taking high doses of vitamin C every day is unlikely to be cured of cancer. Nevertheless, it is possible to raise vitamin C blood levels sufficiently, using oral doses, to kill cancer cells. Such high blood levels can be maintained for years and may inhibit cancer growth.

The vitamin C intake required to maintain maximum blood levels is in the region of 20 grams per day, for a healthy young adult. These doses and levels may be higher in a person with cancer. To achieve steady blood levels, the vitamin C should be split and taken at regular intervals of four hours or less. Since individual vitamin C requirements vary from person to person, Dr Robert Cathcart developed a way of determining the amount that is likely to be effective. This approach is called titrating to bowel tolerance.

Large doses of vitamin C can induce diarrhoea, if taken too quickly. Cathcart suggests increasing the dose gradually, in a series of steps. A person could, for example, take one extra gram each day, until they start to get loose stools. When bowel tolerance is reached, the person reduces the dose by one gram. Since bowel tolerance varies, it helpful for people to keep trying to increase the dose, to try and stay just below their present, individual bowel tolerance. In this way, people can maintain the maximum blood level of vitamin C for a prolonged period.

Notably, there appears to be a relationship between bowel tolerance levels of vitamin C and carbohydrate intake. Sugar inhibits vitamin C uptake. High levels of vitamin C are far more effective with a low carbohydrate diet. This factor may have masked the effectiveness of vitamin C in clinical trials in the overfed western world.

It is important to take these high doses of vitamin C in divided doses, because vitamin C passes through the body quickly. Ideally, this might mean taking, say, a 2 gram dose every hour of the day. However, this dose interval could be impractical, so people might elect to take several grams at 3-4 hourly intervals. Vitamin C at these high doses is rapidly lost from the blood and excreted.[b]

---

[b] People taking high doses of vitamin C should consider supplementing with magnesium citrate (200-400mg per day) to avoid the slight (theoretical) risk of oxalate kidney stones [J Urol. 1997 Dec;158(6):2069-2073].

Recently, a new form of vitamin C has become generally available. Liposomal vitamin C provides improved absorption of high doses than standard forms, when taken orally. The vitamin C is contained in microscopic balls of a fat, called lecithin.[c] This form of oral vitamin C allows much higher blood levels to be maintained.

Preliminary experiments suggest that liposomal vitamin C allows subjects to reach twice the levels obtainable with standard vitamin C tablets. In experiments conducted in the UK, at the Biolab Medical Unit, London, we have been able to show that levels of vitamin C in blood plasma can be maintained at exceptionally high levels.[d]

In this context, if the additional cost of this form of vitamin C is not prohibitive, we recommend its use. It could increase the effectiveness of oral vitamin C as a cancer treatment. The downside is that liposomal vitamin C is comparatively expensive, and sources are currently limited.

Redox cycling

Vitamin C is best known as an antioxidant or reducing agent. However, it can also act in the opposite way, as an oxidant. When acting as an antioxidant, each vitamin C molecule has two electrons, which it donates to neutralise free radicals. However, if it later regains the two electrons, it is acting as an oxidant. Under certain conditions, vitamin C can repeatedly gain and lose electrons, in a process known as a redox cycle. When this happens, hydrogen peroxide, a powerful oxidant, is produced.

As chance would have it, the conditions for such redox cycling to occur exist within tumours.[e] Cancers tend to accumulate free iron and copper, which help them maintain the oxidising state they need to divide and grow. Copper and iron can each react with vitamin C, generating hydrogen peroxide. This kind of reaction is called a Fenton reaction, after Henry Fenton, an English chemist who discovered it in 1893.

---

[c] The lecithin, or phospholipid, coat in commercial liposomes is usually phosphatidylcholine.

[d] Using liposomal vitamin C, we have measured sustained levels of over 400 µM/L in blood plasma, and higher levels may be possible (500-600 µM/L). Previously, the plasma maximum for oral vitamin C was assumed to be 220 µM/L.

[e] It is not really chance. Cancers depend on creating an oxidative state for cell division. Those cells that stop producing catalase, or other effective antioxidant enzymes, have a survival advantage, since they can divide more rapidly.

Fenton reactions, involving metals like copper, generate hydrogen peroxide and other damaging free radicals. Healthy cells keep iron and copper bound to other molecules, so they do not join in a Fenton reaction and generate hydrogen peroxide. Cancer cells are unable to protect themselves in this way, so are damaged by the results of the Fenton reaction.

Healthy cells contain low levels of hydrogen peroxide, which they use for cell signalling and for control of cell division and growth. They also contain powerful antioxidant enzymes, such as catalase, that can break down hydrogen peroxide, harmlessly, to oxygen and water.

In cancer cells, the antioxidant enzyme system is damaged. In particular, cancer cells often do not contain catalase. Thus, malignant cells are unable to defend themselves against the hydrogen peroxide and free radicals produced by massive doses of vitamin C. Consequently, massive doses of vitamin C can kill cancer cells, while improving the health of ordinary tissues.

Vitamin C in sufficiently high doses kills cancer cells and leaves healthy cells unharmed. Taken alone, vitamin C is a weak anticancer agent. Intravenous doses are effective. Massive oral doses can provide a continuous anticancer pressure, inhibiting tumour growth.

Lipoic acid

'Faced with the choice between changing one's mind and proving there is
no need to do so, almost everybody gets busy on the proof.'
John Kenneth Galbraith

If vitamin C were the only substance that could kill cancer cells while
not harming the body, it would be an interesting and useful aid to
conventional treatment. However, despite offering a major breakthrough
in cancer therapy, vitamin C on its own is not enough. Fortunately, there
are other safe anticancer substances. One that has been investigated is
alpha-lipoic acid. This shares many of the properties of vitamin C;
furthermore, the two work well together.

A powerful antioxidant

Alpha-lipoic acid is a powerful antioxidant that is soluble in both
water and fat. Together with vitamin C, it provides a solid base of
antioxidant protection. Like vitamin C, it passes through the body rapidly,
which means that frequent doses are needed to raise blood levels
consistently.

Alpha-lipoic acid is a more powerful antioxidant than vitamin C.
Indeed, it is one of the most powerful, small antioxidants in the body.
Unlike vitamin C, however, it needs to be reduced (given electrons)
before the body can make full use of its antioxidant power. In contrast,
vitamin C comes with 'free' electrons, which can be donated to the body.

The combination of alpha-lipoic acid and vitamin C is particularly
powerful. The free antioxidant electrons from high dose vitamin C
generate a reducing environment, in which alpha-lipoic acid acts as a
strong antioxidant. The two substances work together to provide
antioxidant support for healthy cells, but kill cancer cells by generating
hydrogen peroxide and other oxidants.[a]

---

[a] Casciari J.J. Riordan N.H. Schmidt T.L. Meng X.L. Jackson J.A. Riordan H.D. (2001)
Cytotoxicity of ascorbate, lipoic acid, and other antioxidants in hollow fibre *in vitro* tumours,
British Journal of Cancer, 84, 11, 1544-1550.

Generating free radicals

Like vitamin C, alpha-lipoic acid generates hydrogen peroxide and free radicals in cancer cells. High doses of alpha-lipoic acid can destroy cancer cells, while leaving healthy cells unharmed. This presents the exciting possibility that a combination of alpha lipoic acid and vitamin C could form a safe, powerful anticancer treatment.

The doses of lipoic acid required for an anticancer effect are relatively high. However, doses at the level of one or more grams appear to be well tolerated. We know of patients who took three grams a day (e.g. 500mg every four hours) for months, with no side effects. Under medical supervision, divided oral doses of alpha-lipoic acid, totalling five or more grams per day, may be taken.

Synergy

In combination, high concentrations of vitamin C and alpha-lipoic acid are more than five times as powerful as vitamin C alone. When combined, they cause greater cancer cell death than if taken separately. This feature is described as synergy: the combination is greater than the sum of the individual effects. Importantly, combination does not seem to increase toxicity.

When discussing vitamin C, we explained that it was a relatively weak anticancer agent and, at best, only partially effective when taken orally.[b] However, the combination of lipoic acid and vitamin C is powerful: it could be expected to kill more types of cancer and provide greater inhibition of tumour growth than either alone. High oral doses of vitamin C and lipoic acid, in combination, may enable cancer patients to live longer, without significant side effects.

Practicality

When taken orally, lipoic acid is not well absorbed, although it is absorbed better when taken on an empty stomach. Like vitamin C, high doses are excreted rapidly, so should be taken in divided doses. As a rule of thumb, people should take alpha-lipoic acid at the same frequency as dynamic flow vitamin C (every three or four hours).

---

[b] Liposomal forms are more effective, providing an intermediate between oral and intravenous doses and are the preferred approach for cancer therapy.

Alpha-lipoic acid comes in two forms, called r-alpha-lipoic acid and s-alpha-lipoic acid. R-alpha-lipoic acid is the 'natural' form, but synthetic supplements contain both types. The r-form is identical to that produced by the body. Ideally, r-alpha-lipoic acid is preferable, as this is absorbed more easily and may enter tumours more effectively. However, r-alpha-lipoic acid is more expensive and slightly harder to obtain. Alpha-lipoic acid is more expensive than vitamin C, but the cost is still extremely low for a potentially effective anticancer agent. The r-alpha lipoic acid form is most likely to be beneficial in cancer.

Alpha lipoic acid can destroy cancer cells and leave healthy cells undamaged. Like vitamin C, it is a 'penicillin for cancer', generating hydrogen peroxide inside cancer cells. When combined with massive doses of vitamin C, it becomes far more effective. Oral doses of r-alpha-lipoic acid and vitamin C may extend the life of terminal cancer patients.

Vitamin K

'We should always assume the disease to be curable, until
its own natures prove it otherwise.' Peter Mere Latham

Given that research has shown vitamin C and alpha-lipoic acid to be
effective anticancer agents, we wondered whether other supplements
might act in this way. Once we started to look, we realised that there are
several other selective anticancer agents. Vitamin K, in particular, is
complementary to vitamin C and can also destroy cancer cells

Vitamin K is best known for its role in blood clotting: deficiency
causes abnormal bleeding. There are several forms of vitamin K,
including K1, K2 and K3. Of these, vitamin K3 has shown the largest
anticancer effect, although K1 and K2 can also be effective.

K3 kills cancer

Vitamin K3 is an uncommon form of vitamin K, with lower vitamin
activity and somewhat increased toxicity. For these reasons, it is not
normally used as a dietary supplement; vitamins K1 and K2 are more
widely available.

Since the structure of vitamin K3 is similar to that of some standard
anticancer drugs, it is not surprising that it can kill cancer cells selectively.
Vitamin K3 is toxic, because it can generate hydrogen peroxide, in a
Fenton reaction. Healthy cells can remove a reasonable excess of
hydrogen peroxide, whereas tumour cells are unable to detoxify it and are
killed.

Synergy

As we described earlier, synergy occurs if the combined effect of two
substances working together is greater than the sum of their individual
effects. Vitamin K3 is far more powerful as an anticancer agent when
combined with vitamin C: compared to its use alone, the combination is
about 30 times as effective. This is because vitamin C drives vitamin K in
a futile redox cycle, generating hydrogen peroxide, which kills cancer
cells.

This same mechanism is found in a related drug, motexafin gadolinium. Researchers are currently conducting clinical trials, and hope this new anticancer drug will have low toxicity. The drug is chemically related to vitamin K3 and works in the same way. Like vitamin K3, motexafin gadolinium works more powerfully when combined with high doses of vitamin C.

Practicality

Vitamin K3 is relatively difficult to obtain and administer. Health food shops do not stock supplements of vitamin K3. However, at least one company has released a vitamin C and K3 mixture, in a single tablet, intended for men with cancer of the prostate.

Vitamin K3 needs to be administered by a physician. The relative toxicity of vitamin K3, compared to lipoic acid, underlies the necessity for clinical monitoring of its use as an anticancer agent. However, the combination of vitamins K3 and C is potentially a powerful anticancer therapy. More importantly, its selective action indicates how easy it is to find anticancer nutrients in the diet. Such substances need to be isolated and taken in higher doses in supplement form to be fully effective.

Vitamin K can kill cancer cells selectively. There are several forms, of which vitamin K3 is the most effective anticancer agent. Its benefits are greatly enhanced by combination with vitamin C.

Natural cancer killers

'Common sense is not so common.' Voltaire

Medical scientists have searched the world for potential anticancer agents, sampling exotic plants from desert cacti to rainforest trees. This might lead us to think that anticancer substances are rare, although occasionally a new treatment may be discovered. In reality, natural, safe, cancer-killing substances are widespread: animals and plants have been developing such defences for hundreds of millions of years.

Over millions of years, multicellular organisms have built up defence mechanisms to prevent renegade cells becoming cancerous. The evolutionary process has selected substances that destroy or slow the growth of cancer, but are harmless to healthy cells. As a result, anticancer agents are common. Kitchen spices, such as turmeric, are full of them. In addition, a wide range of food supplements will kill or slow the growth of cancer cells; examples are listed at the end of this chapter.

Why don't doctors use them?

Natural anticancer agents are not widely used by the medical profession, most of whom are unaware of their potential. The most likely explanation for this ignorance is that the search for anticancer agents, together with their preparation into effective medications, is driven by the pharmaceutical industry.

Drug companies are interested in substances that can be patented, to protect future profits. The profit from drugs, including anticancer treatments, is enormous: thousands of dollars per patient per year. In terms of business profitability, no other sector comes close.[c] By contrast, natural substances, such as vitamins, cannot be patented. This means that, however effective they may be, they cannot be used to generate huge profits. In particular, a nutritional substance such as vitamin K will not generate the profits of a drug such as motexafin gadolinium, even though both work in a similar way. From a commercial drug company viewpoint, natural anticancer agents are unwelcome competition.

---

[c] Reported by Dr Marcia Angell and was true for the decade up to 2002: since 2003, mining/oil and banking have been very profitable also.

An extensive marketing and public relations machine exists to service the pharmaceutical industry; it protects their profits by activities such as promoting patented drugs, lobbying politicians, funding patient pressure groups, and disparaging alternatives in the media. The aim of this effort is to ensure that doctors know about expensive new drugs, and that patients demand them.

Why no large-scale clinical trials?

In the face of the pharmaceutical industry's financial dominance, well-intentioned scientists and physicians are powerless. Even if they wanted to test natural treatments, they would be unlikely to get funding. It costs millions of dollars to fund clinical trials of cancer treatments. This places severe restrictions on scientists wishing to investigate new therapies.

Many conventional medical scientists have close links to drug companies, who provide substantial research funds. Ideas that could fundamentally change the status quo could also threaten a scientist's career prospects. Since drug companies are driven by profits, there is no reason for them to test natural anticancer substances, unless they are attempting to discredit them.

Nutritional medicine

Although superior in terms of marketing, drug companies are at a disadvantage when it comes to discovering new anticancer agents. Current knowledge of the disease is inadequate, researchers are restricted by the need to obtain patents, and the time available to produce the next drug is limited. It may take decades to investigate a new substance; meanwhile, the patent on the previous one will be running out.

By comparison, evolution has had hundreds of millions of years to develop effective therapies. Natural selection has favoured the most successful. Any animal or plant that produces a safe anticancer agent has an evolutionary advantage. Multicellular creatures have had a billion years of selection pressure to develop methods for preventing cancer growth. It is not surprising that nutritional supplements, arising from evolutionary developments, can kill cancer cells with fewer side effects than anticancer drugs. The myth that nutritional supplements are of little value to health is misplaced and is not based on good scientific data.

Prevention

It is widely accepted that substances in food can protect people from cancer. Both conventional and nutritional medicine offer guidelines for cancer prevention. The presence of numerous substances in plants that can help prevent cancer is uncontroversial, as is the idea that antioxidants might hold the key to cancer prevention.

Anticancer agents in food are typically present in small amounts. They may be sufficient to inhibit tumour growth in the source plant, but are diluted when they enter the body. Eating 200 grams of a vegetable will not raise the level of a substance much in a 70 kilogram body. Supplements provide larger and more consistent doses. Turmeric supplements may contain concentrations of curcumin twenty times that in the original spice, for example. A one gram tablet is equivalent to 20 grams of the raw dried spice; it would be hard to consume an equivalent amount by eating curry.

Therapy

If plants contain substances that help prevent cancer, these might form the basis of treatments. Furthermore, if a substance could be isolated and concentrated, it could be given in higher doses, which may be more beneficial. Therapeutic doses generally require supplements, not just eating more vegetables. However, there are risks to this approach: increasing the dose of a substance could cause side effects, which were not apparent when consuming lower intakes of the original plant.

It is relatively easy to exclude any acutely toxic substances, as the risk of toxicity from nutrients is low. There are very few recorded deaths from vitamin overdose in the United States; a typical person is in greater risk of being struck by a lightning bolt. However, even with a safe substance, treatment can have its dangers. One risk with the use of intravenous vitamin C is that it can be too effective. If it destroys a tumour too quickly, the patient can go into toxic shock. For this reason, nutritional treatment of cancer requires medical supervision.

Often, two nutritional substances work together to destroy cancer more effectively; we have seen this with vitamin C and alpha-lipoic acid. However, some natural anticancer agents may counteract the effects of others. For example, antioxidants may neutralise the oxidative, anticancer action of vitamin C. People wishing to treat or prevent cancer should choose their supplements carefully, and only take those likely to be synergistic in killing cancer or preventing its growth.

Large numbers of substances that can kill cancer cells exist and are commonly found in vegetables and spices. These substances are often safe, even in large intakes. Such safe anticancer agents may provide the future treatment of cancer.

Preventing cancer
(Phase 0 therapy)

The following nutritional regime is aimed at preventing cancer. Additional cancer prevention advice, such as not smoking tobacco or, if female, avoiding the contraceptive pill, should also be followed.

Good nutrition is an accepted part of cancer prevention. In particular, a low carbohydrate diet with a high intake of vegetables could be beneficial. Antioxidant supplementation may reduce the risk of developing cancer.

- Vitamin C (as L-ascorbic acid) - dynamic flow level, half a gram or more, 5/6 times a day

- R-alpha-lipoic acid - 50-100mg, twice daily

- Vitamin D3 - 1000 iu/day

- Selenium - 200 μG/day

- Absorbable magnesium - 200-400mg/day as magnesium citrate or magnesium chelate

- Vitamin E - 400 iu/day, preferably mixed natural tocopherols and tocotrienols

- Good general nutritional supplement support (e.g. multivitamins and minerals)

- Cut down on sugars (e.g. no sugar in tea or coffee), cakes and biscuits

- Low carbohydrate diet

- Choose colourful, low carbohydrate vegetables (containing antioxidants)

Minor modifications to the diet can produce a reduction in cancer risk.

Remission therapy

(Phase 1 treatment)

Following apparently successful treatment, patients have a dilemma. Do they consider themselves cured of the disease, in which case an optimal diet of antioxidants would be appropriate; or do they consider themselves to have some remaining cancer cells, in which case they would require a restricted diet to inhibit future growth? Conservatively, we assume that some cancer cells remain, even if the person is in remission. People at higher risk of cancer may choose this approach for prevention, rather than Phase 0.

- Vitamin C (as L-ascorbic acid) - dynamic flow level, at least 1 gram with each meal, preferably >10g per day.

- R-alpha-lipoic acid - 100 mg with each gram of vitamin C

- Vitamin D3 - 2500iu/day

- Selenium - 200 µG/day (as methylselenocysteine)

- Absorbable magnesium - 200-400mg/day as magnesium citrate or magnesium chelate

- No additional supplements

- Low carbohydrate diet, no sugar

- Lots of fresh vegetables and fruit (raw): choose colourful, low carbohydrate vegetables

Cooked starchy vegetables, such as potatoes, are a source of protein and glucose. A 'healthy' baked potato may release more sugar to the body than an equivalent sized chocolate bar. It is important to lower sugar intake, from all sources. The availability of sugar in foods can be estimated from books on glycaemic index (GI) or glycaemic load (GL).[d] Lowering sugar intake is particularly difficult as people crave sweet food. Fortunately, the palate responds to adjustments; sugared tea can taste horrible once people become accustomed to unsweetened beverages.

---

[d] There are many books on low carbohydrate and low GI diets, for example: Brand-Miller J. Foster-Powell K. McMillan-Price J. (2005) The Low GI Diet Revolution: The Definitive Science-Based Weight Loss Plan, Marlowe & Company.

Minimal therapy
(Phase 2 treatment)

A person with a slow-growing cancer, or who is unable to make major changes to their lifestyle, might opt for minimal dietary change. Perhaps the patient does not really believe in nutritional medicine, but is willing to make limited adjustments. The main change is increased vitamin C intake and lower carbohydrates.

- Vitamin C (as L-ascorbic acid) - dynamic flow level, at least 1g with each meal, preferably >10g per day. Liposomal formulations should be considered and are recommended for higher doses.

- R-alpha-lipoic acid - 100 mg with each gram of vitamin C

- Vitamin D3 - 4000 iu/day

- Selenium - 400 μG/day (as methylselenocysteine)

- Absorbable magnesium - 200-400mg/day as magnesium citrate or magnesium chelate

- No additional supplements

- Low carbohydrate diet

- No sugar

- Lots of fresh raw vegetables and fruit.

As the cancer is more threatening, the diet becomes more restrictive. The carbohydrate is reduced further, as is the total calorie intake. The easiest way to achieve this is a diet based around raw vegetables and fruit.

Easy therapy

(Phase 3 treatment)

Some patients may wish to move forward with nutritional treatment but are not willing to fully commit to a strictly controlled diet. If, after trying this phase, monitoring shows that the growth of cancer has not slowed, move to Phase 4 therapy.

- Vitamin C (as L-ascorbic acid) - dynamic flow level, at least 2g with each meal, preferably >10g per day. Close to bowel tolerance. Liposomal formulations are preferred with higher intakes.

- R-alpha-lipoic acid - 100-200mg with each gram of vitamin C

- Vitamin D3 - 4000 iu/day

- Selenium - 400-600 μG/day (as methylselenocysteine)

- Absorbable magnesium – 400-800mg/day as magnesium citrate or magnesium chelate

- No additional supplements

- Low-carbohydrate and low calorie diet

- No sugar

- Lots of fresh raw vegetables

In this phase, vitamin C level approach bowel tolerance. Liposomal formulations increase blood levels and may allow a greater daily intake. The r-alpha-lipoic acid intake is similarly increased in this therapeutic phase. The levels of selenium are high and a few sensitive people may experience minor side effects (described later) which resolve if the dose is lowered.

Standard therapy

(Phase 4 treatment)

This would be considered a standard approach for most cancer patients who are not in the final stages of the disease. If, after trying this phase, monitoring shows that the growth of cancer has not slowed, move to Phase 5 therapy.

- Vitamin C (as L-ascorbic acid) - dynamic flow level, at least 3g five or six times each day, providing a daily total of 20g or more. (> 90% bowel tolerance).
  Liposomal formulations are highly recommended.

- R-alpha-lipoic acid - 200-500mg with each dose of vitamin C (up to 5g total oral intake)

- Vitamin D3 - 4000 iu/day

- Selenium - 800 μG/day (as methylselenocysteine)

- Absorbable magnesium – 400-2500mg/day as magnesium citrate or magnesium chelate

- No additional supplements

- Very low carbohydrate and low calorie diet

- Lots of fresh raw vegetables

This is a severe dietary restriction, involving low calories and, in particular, reduced intake of carbohydrates and proteins. Essentially, it corresponds to severe dietary restriction with the highest tolerated intakes of vitamin C and r-alpha-lipoic acid.

The level of selenium intake corresponds to the United States government's no observed adverse effect level (NOAEL), and is the maximum intake considered safe of any side effects.

Aggressive oral therapy
(Phase 5 treatment)

This is an aggressive oral therapy for cancer. It is appropriate for people in the latter stages of the disease. However, patients in earlier stages may choose a similar approach, to maximise the chances of a longer symptom-free life. If monitoring shows the treatment to be ineffective, move to next stage (Phase 6).

- Vitamin C (as L-ascorbic acid) – maximum dynamic flow level, at least 3g five or six times each day, providing a daily total of 20g or more. (> 90% bowel tolerance). Liposomal formulations are highly recommended.

- R-alpha-lipoic acid - 200-500mg with each dose of vitamin C (up to 5g total oral intake)

- Vitamin D3 - 4000 iu/day

- Selenium - consider 1-3mg per day, (as methylselenocysteine) under strict medical supervision

- Absorbable magnesium – 400-2500mg/day as magnesium citrate or magnesium chelate

- Consider copper gluconate, say 2mg, twice per day

- No additional supplements

- Diet largely of raw fresh vegetables, with no carbohydrates (<25g carbs per day)

This level of selenium is potentially toxic and should not be undertaken without physician guidance, support and monitoring.[a] It equates to an intensive chemotherapy. People concerned about the possibility of selenium toxicity can reduce the intake to the no observed adverse effect level (800 µG/day) or below. This value has an uncertainty factor of two, based on a 55 Kg adult, indicating that doses of 1600 µG/day are safe in the long term.

---

[a] Your doctor will monitor for possible symptoms of toxicity including fingernail weakening, garlic odour of breath and sweat, hair loss, irritability, itching of skin, metallic taste, nausea and vomiting, unusual tiredness and weakness.

Intensive therapy
(Phase 6 treatment)

This therapy uses intravenous treatment in combination with oral therapy. The intravenous treatment can be used to shrink the tumour early on, or can be employed with the onset of symptoms. A typical cycle of intravenous treatment would be three infusions of 75 -100g of sodium ascorbate (perhaps with r-alpha-lipoic acid or vitamin K3) three times per week, for five weeks.

- Vitamin C (as L-ascorbic acid) – maximum dynamic flow level, at least 3g five or six times each day, providing a daily total of 20g or more. (> 90% bowel tolerance) Liposomal formulations are highly recommended.

- R-alpha-lipoic acid - 200-500mg with each dose of vitamin C (up to 5g total oral intake).

- Vitamin D3 - 4000 iu/day

- Selenium[b] - 1-3mg per day (as methylselenocysteine) under strict medical supervision

- Absorbable magnesium – 400-2500mg/day as magnesium citrate or magnesium chelate

- Copper gluconate, ~ 2mg, twice per day

- Oral vitamin K3 should be considered

- Introduce IV vitamin C therapy, combined with lipoic acid or vitamin K3.

- No additional supplements

- Raw vegetable diet, minimal carbohydrates

This approach combines a strict low carbohydrate and calorie diet with maximum intakes of active supplements. This can be used in conjunction with intravenous doses of sodium ascorbate, which need to be provided by a suitably qualified physician.

---

[b] A note on selenium toxicity is provided on the previous page.

Does this therapy work?

An American scientist visited the great Nobel Prize-winning physicist, Niels Bohr, in Copenhagen. He was astounded to find a lucky horseshoe nailed to the wall. The scientist asked, with a nervous laugh, 'Surely, Professor Bohr, you don't believe that horseshoe will bring you good luck?' Bohr laughed. 'Not at all, I am scarcely likely to believe in such foolish nonsense. They tell me it works whether you believe in it or not!'

There are many books on what to eat if you have cancer. As far as we can tell, most rely more on wishful thinking than scientific evidence. In contrast, this book presents an approach to the nutritional treatment of cancer that is consistent with available scientific facts.

Scientific evidence suggests that oral redox therapy, as described in this book, can prolong the life of cancer patients. This has not been confirmed by clinical trials in humans, for the simple reason that such trials have not yet been performed. We are keen to see such trials carried out as soon as possible.

Although experiments on the cancer-killing actions of vitamin C were published in 1969, medical science has not yet investigated the potential of this treatment properly. Dr Linus Pauling and Dr Ewan Cameron published clinical trials, which suggested that cancer patients treated with intravenous vitamin C could live 5-6 times longer than expected. Similar degrees of life extension have been confirmed by other scientists, including Dr Abram Hoffer.

Other clinical trials, notably those performed by the Mayo clinic, have failed to confirm these results. The Mayo Clinic trials have been heavily criticised, however. Perhaps the most telling criticism is that not one experimental patient died while taking vitamin C. It is irrational to suggest the results of such an experiment to test increased lifespan were negative, if not a single patient died while on the continuous treatment.

Vitamin C alone, even at high doses, is probably not sufficient to treat cancer. The action of massive doses of vitamin C is, however, increased if carbohydrate intake is low. When taken in combination with other nutritional substances and lifestyle changes, redox therapy, which includes vitamin C, may allow some cancer patients to live a normal lifespan. For further information, our review of the scientific literature is described in our two recent books. These provide solid scientific support for the idea that people with cancer can live longer if they modify their diets and take appropriate supplements.

Our recent book, *Cancer: Nutrition and Survival*, gave a biological overview of the disease and explained the potential for redox therapy. The aim of the present book is to explain more clearly how redox therapy might be undertaken. It is also intended as a guide for scientists, who may wish to undertake research on the effects of redox therapy and selective malnutrition on cancer and its survivability.

The substances discussed in this book have low toxicity. With appropriate medical guidance they can be used safely by cancer patients. Indeed, the suggestions boil down to a low carbohydrate and protein diet, with nutritional supplements. Equivalent oral intakes of vitamin C have been taken by numerous individuals without harm, for decades. The doses of other supplements are quite high, but have not been associated with major side effects. The exception is selenium. While the doses indicated for therapy phases 5 and 6 are higher than the no adverse effect level, they are within the range already studied for cancer treatment; any side effects that might occur can be picked up by clinical monitoring and the dose reduced.

Dr Len Noriega, one of the scientists we asked to review the book before publication, is an expert in decision sciences. Dr Noriega has a personal interest in cancer, having undergone chemotherapy himself. He described our approach as a 'no-brainer' option for terminal patients. Nutritional therapy has a high benefit to risk ratio. The benefits, although not fully explored in clinical trials, may be large. The therapy is relatively safe and inexpensive, with little risk.

Terminal patients for whom no effective conventional treatment is available could usefully consider this option. The alternatives are either to wait to die without hope, or to continue, possibly decades longer, with the hope of survival and a reasonable quality of life.

The efficacy of this approach and related questions might be clarified by well-designed clinical trials in a relatively short period of time. However, such trials are long overdue and, while we wait, people are dying.

As the distinguished scientist and surgeon John Hunter advised Edward Jenner, pioneer of vaccination, in 1775, 'I think your solution is just, but why think? Why not try the experiment?'

Appendix I
Books on nutrition for cancer

There are several widely available books on antioxidant nutrition, suitable for healthy people wanting to avoid cancer. The general aim is a diet rich in antioxidants and low in carbohydrates. However, such supernutrition is not appropriate for people with cancer, who need fewer nutrients, minimal carbohydrates, and specific anticancer supplements.

Linus Pauling (2006) *How to live longer and feel better*, Oregon State University Press. A classic book on nutrition and health.

Andrew Saul (2005) *Fire Your Doctor! How to Be Independently Healthy*, Basic Health Publications. An entertaining and informative book on nutrition and health.

Andrew Saul (2003) *Doctor Yourself: Natural Healing That Works*, Basic Health Publications. Andrew Saul switches the viewpoint from disease care to health care.

Abram Hoffer (1998) *Putting It All Together: The New Orthomolecular Nutrition*, McGraw-Hill. Dr Hoffer presents decades of experience in nutritional medicine.

Eydie Mae Hunsberger (1992) *How I Conquered Cancer Naturally*, Avery. A book by a woman who tracked down an approach to treating cancer using a simple vegetable diet, inspiring scientists to look more carefully at the issues.

Ann Wigmore (1985) *The Wheatgrass Book: How to Grow and Use Wheatgrass to Maximize Your Health and Vitality*, Avery, presents the idea that a diet of raw vegetables can prolong life for cancer patients. (NB: in our opinion, juicing should be avoided as it releases nutrients).

Steve Hickey and Hilary Roberts (2005) *Cancer: Nutrition and Survival*, Lulu Press. Our previous book on cancer provides the scientific background for this book. It explains cancer as an evolutionary process and shows how antioxidants can be used to kill cancer cells selectively.

Appendix 2
Specific anticancer nutrients

Large numbers of food substances are known to be powerful anticancer agents, with little risk; we list a short selection here. Individual substances have their own supporters and detractors. We include this section only to give an indication of the massive, untapped potential of nutritional therapy in cancer.

Some of these substances may act synergistically, working more effectively when used in combination. In other cases, sets of substances may be antagonistic; for example, some antioxidants may be contraindicated if on vitamin C therapy, as they may inhibit the desired pro-oxidant damage to tumour cells.

In this section, we mention a few, selective anticancer agents that are available as food supplements. Our list does not include all possible substances; it merely gives an idea of the range. Unfortunately, many doctors are not aware of the actions of substances on this list, suggesting that cancer research is failing to investigate these potentially life-saving therapies.

Broccoli, Brussels sprouts and cabbage

Cruciferous plants, such as broccoli, sprouts and cabbage, contain powerful and relatively safe anticancer agents.[a] In test tube experiments, these substances killed prostate, breast and cervical cancer cells. Animal studies support these findings, but researchers have not conducted many trials. Two of the active substances, I3C and DIM, are available as dietary supplements.

Another class of anticancer agent found in cruciferous vegetables, isothiocyanates, is not currently available in supplement form. Broccoli sprouts (like bean sprouts, but grown from broccoli seeds) contain isothiocyanates, such as sulforaphane, which prevent cancer growth and kill cancer cells. There are several different substances in this group, which have not been fully investigated for anticancer activity.

---

[a] Indole-3-carbinol (I3C) and 3,3'-diindolylmethane (DIM) are released from cruciferous vegetables in the diet and are available as nutritional supplements.

Carotenoids

The carotenoids, such as beta carotene, possess some antioxidant activity. In particular, lycopene, from tomatoes, has been associated with a reduction in prostate cancer. However, a controversial study of beta carotene suggested that it could increase the incidence of lung cancer in smokers. A possible explanation for this is that beta carotene would not act as an antioxidant in tissues that are subject to continued insult, such as smokers' lungs. For this reason, people using beta carotene as an antioxidant should also supplement with high levels of vitamin C.

Chili pepper

Capsaicin, the substance which makes chili peppers taste hot, can slow the growth of prostate cancer and other tumours, and cause cancer cells to commit suicide by apoptosis. Supplements of capsaicin are widely available. Chili peppers contain several other similar compounds, which await testing for anticancer activity.[b]

Coenzyme Q10

Coenzyme Q10 has a similar chemical structure to vitamin K3 and, in combination with vitamin C, may act as a selective anticancer agent. However, there is insufficient data to confirm this suggestion with confidence. Coenzyme Q10 is a major, fat-soluble antioxidant. It is made in the body and also consumed in the diet. Q10 or similar molecules are found in most animal and plant cells. Its alternative name, ubiquinone, refers to its ubiquitous nature and the fact that, like vitamin K, it is a quinone.

Q10 is involved in the production of energy within cells, and acts as an antioxidant in cell membranes. People taking statin drugs to lower cholesterol are less able to make coenzyme Q10 and may require daily supplements. Beta blockers, taken for high blood pressure, can also deplete Q10. Q10 offers many health benefits and, as a principal antioxidant, should be one of the first supplements considered by a person wishing to prevent cancer.

---

[b] Chili peppers also include dihydrocapsaicin and several minor capsaicinoids, including nordihydrocapsaicin, homodihydrocapsaicin, and homocapsaicin.

Copper

Copper is a metal that, like iron, can drive a Fenton reaction. In combination with vitamin C and/or lipoic acid this can result in the generation of hydrogen peroxide, which is lethal to cancer cells. Tumours may concentrate copper and are more sensitive to the effects of the hydrogen peroxide it produces. Supplements, such as copper gluconate, can be considered to help drive redox therapy.

Garlic

Garlic is a rich source of sulphur-containing compounds, which have potential to prevent and treat disease. Crushing or chopping garlic releases allicin. Allicin rapidly breaks down to form a variety of substances. The quality and the number of active compounds in garlic supplements and preparations is highly variable. Quality is an essential consideration when garlic is considered for cancer prevention or treatment.

Studies of human populations suggest that high intakes of garlic and related vegetables, such as onion, may help protect against gastric and colorectal cancer. Garlic is a good source of selenium compounds, which may explain some of its anticancer effect.

Studies suggest that garlic and its components can inhibit cancer. The effects of garlic are quite broad, based on test tube, animal and dietary studies in humans. At high concentrations, some of the components of garlic will kill cancer cells and may be useful in treatment.[c]

Side effects of garlic include breath odour. Occasionally, allergic reactions and other disorders can occur. While garlic supplementation is considered safe, the massive doses required for cancer therapy require medical supervision.

Ginger

Ginger is one of a family of plants that contain several selective anticancer agents. Substances in ginger can slow cancer growth and kill cancer cells. It has been proposed as a potential therapy for bowel and ovarian cancer, for example. Ginger is generally regarded as safe, but contains substances that can selectively kill cancer cells.

---

[c] Garlic contains ajoene, allicin, diallyl disulfide and diallyl sulphide, S-allylcysteine, S-allylmercaptocysteine and other substances that can kill cancer cells.

Grape seed extract

Grape seed extract is a powerful antioxidant found in the seeds of grapes, especially red ones. Blueberries and pine bark extract contain similar antioxidants.[d] Grape seed extract may support the antioxidant effects of vitamin C. In particular, it has similar properties in preventing abnormal growth and destroying cancer cells, while not harming healthy cells.

Graviola

Graviola is a small evergreen tree, with large, glossy dark green leaves. Its large fruit is yellow-green in colour, with white flesh inside. Graviola grows in the warmest tropical areas in South and North America, including the Amazon. The fruit is sold in local markets in the tropics. Graviola is claimed to be a powerful anticancer agent because it contains substances with antitumour, antiparasitic, insecticidal, and antimicrobial activities.[e] The custard-apple family, to which it belongs, has not been well studied and it is too early to be certain that this will be a useful anticancer agent.

IP6

Laboratory and animal experiments suggest that inositol hexaphosphate (IP6), a sugar phosphate, can be an effective treatment for cancer. It acts by binding and removing iron. Iron is potentially an oxidant and is a growth factor for some cancers. When iron is in short supply, tumour growth is inhibited. IP6 may prevent cancer by acting as an antioxidant. When IP6 binds iron, the resulting reducing state makes cancer cells less able to proliferate and grow.[f]

Paradoxically, IP6 could inhibit the anti-cancer action of vitamin C. Vitamin C based redox therapy works in the opposite way to IP6: it kills cancer cells by making them more oxidising. When iron and vitamin C combine, they generate hydrogen peroxide in cancer cells. However, if the iron has been removed by IP6, this reaction may be prevented.

---

[d] Proanthocyanidins.

[e] Annonaceous acetogenins.

[f] A reducing state is the opposite of an oxidising state. In a reducing environment, there are 'spare' electrons, to neutralise free radicals. In an oxidising environment, electrons get 'stolen', creating damaging free radicals.

Until we know more about the interactions between redox therapy and IP6, the choice seems to be either IP6 or vitamin C, but not both. IP6 could be useful to slow progression or prevent relapse in people who may have been cured, perhaps by surgery. However, clinical evidence is not available, as studies have not been conducted.

Iron

Iron drives Fenton reactions and can be used in combination with vitamin C and lipoic acid. However, tumours often concentrate iron and use it as a growth factor. For this reason, supplementing vitamin C based therapy with copper, rather than iron, may be more effective.

Laetrile

Laetrile is a substance derived from apricot seeds. It has been suggested that laetrile, or the similar compound amygdalin, has selective anticancer activity. However, studies are inconclusive and, taken orally, laetrile could be poisonous. More research is needed to determine the relative costs and benefits of laetrile, as a therapy for cancer. It is included here for completeness. Laetrile has a chequered history, based on prejudice rather than appropriate scientific investigation.

Luteolin

Luteolin is a citrus bioflavonoid, which occurs naturally in parsley, thyme and peppermint, among others. Luteolin is an antioxidant, which also promotes carbohydrate metabolism. It has been shown to inhibit several cancers, including colon and prostate cancer. It can induce apoptosis in cancer cells, and inhibits insulin-like growth factor receptors, which are necessary for prostate cancer growth.

Lycopene

Tomatoes contain lycopene, which can slow cancer growth and kill cancer cells. Lycopene is an antioxidant, which may prevent several forms of cancer, including stomach, rectal, prostate, lung and breast cancer.

Quercetin

Quercetin is a widespread dietary bioflavonoid. It may prevent cancer and could also be an effective treatment. When taken orally, at high doses, quercetin is considered safe.

Oral absorption used to be thought to be poor in humans, but this appears to have been overstated. In human studies, blood concentration has been claimed to be too low to kill cancer cells; however, this may reflect inadequate intakes. In test tube studies, quercetin inhibits the growth of cancer cells. In animal studies, it has been shown to lead to an extended life-span.

Resveratrol

Resveratrol is an antioxidant, found in red grapes, red wine, peanuts, and some berries. Scientists have claimed that the 'French paradox' (according to which French people have a low incidence of heart disease, despite a diet allegedly rich in saturated fats) may be explained by their consumption of resveratrol. Resveratrol belongs to a class of anticancer nutrients called salvestrols.

Scientists have shown that resveratrol can inhibit the growth of cancer cells in culture and in animal models. In addition, it may boost the action of other anticancer nutrients, such as quercetin.

Rutin

Rutin is a citrus flavonoid, a compound of quercetin and a disaccharide, rutinose. Found in buckwheat, among other sources, it acts as an antioxidant. Some researchers have suggested that rutin can help prevent cancers.

Like IP6, rutin may bond with iron in such a way as to inhibit Fenton reactions, which would make it unsuitable for use in combination with vitamin C / redox therapy.

Selenium

Selenium is a mineral that comes in several forms. It is an essential trace element, which acts as a powerful antioxidant in the body, and supports the activity of vitamin E. Animal studies have shown that high level supplementation with selenium reduces the incidence of cancer. Human studies in different countries suggest that selenium has a protective effect against cancer, particularly for undernourished individuals. It is likely to prove to be one of the most important anticancer agents.

Selenium may reduce the overall incidence and mortality of cancer, particularly liver, prostate, colorectal, and lung cancers. Individuals with the lowest selenium status appear to obtain the greatest benefit from supplementation.[g]

Selenium is known to kill cancer cells. At high doses, its anticancer action depends on its role as a pro-oxidant. Scientists have suggested that, because of its low toxicity, it could eventually become the drug of choice for treatment of many cancers, including leukaemia. Healthy cells, which possess intact antioxidant defences, are resistant to selenium. Selenium enhances the action of some conventional anticancer drugs, while reducing their side effects.

Care is needed, as selenium poisoning is occasionally reported. Although selenium is an essential dietary requirement, high doses can be toxic. The 'no observed adverse effect' level is 800 micrograms per day. In a recent study, 16 men with prostate cancer were given 3200 micrograms a day for a year, with no serious toxicities. Doses of up to about 6mg (6000 micrograms) per day have been proposed for treatment of cancer.

Dr Abram Hoffer suggests that, for short intervals, doses of 5-10mg may act as a form of chemotherapy, with associated side effects. If taken for an extended period, this level could result in selenium accumulation and side effects. However, the cost-effectiveness and relatively low toxicity of selenium have been used to support its consideration as an anticancer therapy.

Silibinin

Silibinin is an antioxidant flavonoid, derived from milk thistle. It may protect against skin and prostate cancer, and studies with mice have shown that it can inhibit the growth of lung cancers. Silibinin may be of use for those cancer patients who wish to use conventional methods rather than, or in conjunction with, nutritional treatments, as it helps prevent the kidney damage caused by many chemotherapeutic drugs.[h]

---

[g] The level of nutritional selenium needed to provide optimal benefits may be that required to maximize the activity of selenoenzymes.

[h] Many antioxidants, such as high dose vitamin C, enhance the effectiveness and limit the side-effects of some forms of conventional chemotherapy.

Turmeric

Turmeric, a yellow curry spice, has powerful anti-inflammatory, antioxidant and anticancer properties. These properties arise from curcumin and related substances in the plant. The turmeric plant is a member of the ginger family and has been used in Indian medicine for centuries. Western medicine has recently started to investigate its remarkable properties. It is used as a food additive and yellow colouring ingredient, in foods such as mustard. It has the additive number E100, which shows that not all food additives are harmful to heath.[i]

Curcumin is a selective anticancer and anti-inflammatory agent. It may prevent cancer growth and kill cancer cells. Defence of the conventional, toxic approach to chemotherapy is made particularly difficult by the existence of spices like turmeric.

Curcumin is recommended as a cancer preventative. It also helps with chronic inflammatory diseases, such as arthritis.

Vitamin A

The anticancer properties of vitamin A and related substances, called retinoids,[j] have been established over the past few decades. In test tube studies, retinoic acid has been found to kill many human cancers. There have been limited trials in human cancer patients and results have been variable. Vitamin A derivatives are not suitable as a single therapy for cancer.

Vitamin B

The well-known vitamin B complex consists of a range of substances.[k] These work better when taken together and multi-B complex formulations are widely available. According to Bruce Ames, Professor of Biochemistry and Molecular Biology at the University of California, deficiencies of B6, B12 and folic acid can cause DNA damage and lead to cancer. People wanting to avoid cancer should consider supplementing

---

[i] Other useful food additives include E300 (ascorbic acid or vitamin C), and E101 (riboflavin or vitamin B2).

[j] Anticancer retinoids include all-trans retinoic acid and 13-cis-retinoic acid (isotretinoin).

[k] Including B1 (thiamine), B2 (riboflavin), B3 (niacin or nicotinamide), B5 (pantothenic acid), B6 (pyridoxine), B12 (cobalamin), B15 (pangamic acid), biotin (also known as coenzyme R or vitamin H), PABA (para-aminobenzoic acid), and folic acid.

with a B vitamin complex. Dr Abram Hoffer has used vitamin B3 (niacin), together with vitamin C, to treat cancer.

Vitamin C

Vitamin C is arguably the most important antioxidant in the diet. It is essential to humans since, unlike most animals, we do not synthesise it in our bodies. Vitamin C is water soluble and passes quickly through the body. For this reason, it should be taken in relatively high doses, at short intervals.

In a healthy person, a minimum dose of 500mg with every meal (4 times a day) should be enough to produce dynamic flow. In dynamic flow, vitamin C flows through the body, donating antioxidant electrons to tissues before it is excreted. At dynamic flow levels, vitamin C can recharge other antioxidants, by supplying them with electrons. Liposomal formulations of vitamin C allow much higher blood levels to be attained.

Vitamin D3

Vitamin D is a powerful cancer preventative supplement and should be part of any diet aimed at reducing cancer risk. The preferred form is vitamin D3 (or cholecalciferol). This vitamin is formed by the action of sunlight on skin. People who avoid the sun to reduce the risk of skin cancer, or to prevent ageing, can become relatively deficient. An adequate provision of Vitamin D can greatly reduce the chance of developing cancer.

Vitamin E

Vitamin E is the outstanding fat-soluble antioxidant in the diet. There are several forms of this vitamin. In the body, natural forms are more effective than synthetic ones. There are two main types of vitamin E: tocopherols and tocotrienols. Natural supplements, which contain a mixture of tocopherols and tocotrienols, are preferable as nutritional supplements.[1] Single kinds of vitamin E, such as alpha tocopherol, are less effective than mixed forms, which contain several components, as the different types have specific biological properties.

---

[1] Synthetic forms are usually racemic (a mixture of left- and right-handed versions), prefixed "dl", as in dl-alpha-tocopherol, whereas the natural forms are the "d" type, such as d-alpha-tocopherol.

Some specific forms of vitamin E, such as D-alpha-tocopherol succinate, are selective anticancer agents, but must be given by injection to be effective. The less common tocotrienol forms of vitamin E may have advantages over the popular tocopherols.

Anticancer agents are available from normal foodstuffs. Isolation of these substances in supplement form provides a generally non-toxic approach to fighting cancer. There are a large number of simple safe substances that can be used to slow the growth of, or destroy, cancer cells.

Appendix 3
Scientific justification

Sadly, we do not expect clinical trials of redox therapy in the near future: there is too much prejudice and politics in cancer research. The most likely way for this treatment to become accepted is if terminal cancer patients to elect to try redox therapy and then live far longer than expected. If enough people do this, with the guidance of their medical professionals, the establishment may begin to take notice.

The Mayo Clinic's well-known clinical trials of vitamin C and cancer were badly designed and conducted. We hope that when new clinical trials are performed, they will be done correctly. Most trials of vitamin C, for example, have used doses that were too small and too infrequent, yielding minimally effective results.

Doctors wishing to follow the scientific argument in detail are recommended to consult the following references:

Hickey S. and Roberts H. (2005) *Cancer: Nutrition and Survival*, Lulu Press. This book provides a review of the current scientific position and contains hundreds of specific background references.

Hickey S. and Roberts H. (2004) *Ascorbate: The Science of Vitamin C*, Lulu Press. A book designed to aid understanding of vitamin C and its role in health and disease, written as a follow-up to the work of Linus Pauling.

Linus Pauling and Ewan Cameron (1993) Vitamin C and Cancer: A Discussion of the Nature, Causes, Prevention, and Treatment of Cancer With Special Reference to the Value of Vitamin C, Camino Books. A classic work arising from the collaboration of a scientific genius and a surgeon.

Abram Hoffer and Linus Pauling (2001) *Vitamin C & Cancer: Discovery, Recovery, Controversy*, Scb Distributors. This book gives continuing results from Dr Abram Hoffer, suggesting that vitamin C supplementation benefits cancer patients.

Hickey S. and Roberts H.J. (2005) Dynamic flow, JOM, 20(4), 237-244. This paper explains why high dose studies of vitamin C have underestimated its beneficial effects.

Hickey S. and Roberts H. (2006) Pharmacokinetics invalidate study, Heart Online, August. A short response, illustrating how vitamin C papers have compounded ignorance of high doses of vitamin C.

Hickey S. (2005) Misleading information on the properties of vitamin C, PLOS Medicine, 2(9), e307. This letter explains why studies claiming vitamin C does not prevent or provide an effective treatment for the common cold are fundamentally flawed.

Hickey S. and Roberts H. (2007) Selfish cells: cancer as microevolution, JOM, in press. In this paper, a microevolutionary model is used to explain how cancer is subject to biological controls and how antioxidant nutrition can prevent its growth.

Gonzalez M.J., Miranda-Massari J.R., Mora E.M., Guzman A., Riordan N.H., Riordan H.D., Casciari J.J., Jackson J.A., Roman-Franco A. (2005) Orthomolecular oncology review: ascorbic acid and cancer 25 years later, Integr Cancer Ther, 4(1), 32-44.

Gonzalez M.J., Miranda-Massari J.R., Mora E.M., Jimenez I.Z., Matos M.I., Riordan H.D., Casciari J.J. Riordan N.H. Rodriguez M.Y.S., Guzman A. (2002) Orthomolecular oncology: a mechanistic view of ascorbate's chemotherapeutic activity, P R Health Sci J, 21(1), 39-41.

Padayatty S.J., Sun H., Wang Y., Riordan H.D., Hewitt S.M., Katz A., Wesley R.A., Levine M. (2004) Vitamin C pharmacokinetics: implications for oral and intravenous use, Ann Intern Med, 140, 533-537.

Casciari J.J., Riordan H.D., Miranda-Massari J.R., Gonzalez M.J. (2005) Effects of high dose ascorbate administration on L-10 tumor growth in guinea pigs, P R Health Sci J, 24(2), 145-150.

Gonzalez M.J., Mora E., Riordan N.H., Riordan H.D., Mojica P. (1998) Rethinking Vitamin C And Cancer: An Update On Nutritional Oncology, Cancer Prevention International, 3, 215-234.

Riordan N.H., Riordan H.D., Jackson J.A., Casciari J.P. (2000) Clinical and experimental experiences with intravenous vitamin C, Journal of Orthomolecular Medicine, 15(4) 201-213.

Murata A., Morishige F., Yamaguchi H. (1982) Prolongation of survival times of terminal cancer patients by administration of large doses of ascorbate, International Journal for Vitamin and Nutrition Research, Supplement, 23, 101-113.

What the words mean

Aerobic: an environment or condition that contains oxygen; organisms able to live only in the presence of air or free oxygen.

Amygdalin: a bitter cyanide-generating extract from the seeds of apricots, plums and bitter almond; claimed by some to be a vitamin (B17), which can destroy cancer.

Anaerobic: an environment or condition which is free of oxygen; an organism that grows in the absence of oxygen.

Anticoagulant: any of a variety of drugs which 'thin the blood', preventing clotting. These drugs, which are used to prevent strokes and thrombosis, often work by blocking the effects of vitamin K. Vitamin K supplements should not be taken when using these drugs.

Antioxidant: substance or action that inhibits or prevents oxidation, lessening the damaging effects of free radicals.

Apoptosis: programmed cell death, the method used by the body to dispose of damaged or superfluous cells.

Ascorbate: vitamin C, an essential antioxidant in the diet.

Bacteria: single-celled organisms that multiply by cell division and can cause disease in humans, plants or animals. Some forms of bacteria are essential to human life.

Benign: non-spreading, not malignant, usually not life-threatening.

Calorie: The amount of heat, or thermal, energy required to raise one gram of water by 1°C at 15°C. The standard unit for energy measurement in nutrition is one kilocalorie or 1,000 calories; confusingly, this is usually abbreviated to calorie.

Cancer: a malignant growth or tumour, caused by abnormal and uncontrolled cell division.

Carbohydrate: an organic molecule, or substance, consisting of a chain of carbon atoms to which hydrogen and oxygen are attached in a ration of two (H) to one (O). Examples include sugars, starches, glycogen and cellulose.

Carotenoid: any of several phytonutrients, which give plants a distinctive yellow, orange or red pigmentation. The most well-known of these is beta carotene, found in carrots, from which the group of chemicals takes its name.

Catalase: a haem-based enzyme, which catalyses the breakdown of hydrogen peroxide into oxygen and water.

Cell: the fundamental unit of life, which is capable of growth and reproduction.

Cellulose: The substance from which plant cell walls are formed. These cell walls make plants difficult to digest, but can be broken down by juicing.

Chemotherapy: the use of chemical agents as a treatment for cancer.

Chromosome: Carriers of genetic information in the cell. A length of intertwined DNA, held together by proteins.

Cruciferous: plants belonging to the genus *brassicacae,* including mustard, cabbage, broccoli and sprouts. Many of these contain isothiocyanates.

Curcumin: An antioxidant, molecular formula $C_{21}H_{20}O_6$, found in the spice turmeric. Curcumin has antioxidant properties and is an effective anticancer agent.

Cytotoxic: Poisonous to cells.

DNA: Deoxyribonucleic acid, the substance in a cell nucleus which encodes genetic information.

Dynamic flow: The model which suggests that in order to maintain optimum levels of vitamin C (and other nutrients with a short half-life) in the body, regular doses spaced at relatively short intervals should be taken, creating a constant flow of the nutrient through the blood-stream.

Electron: A negatively-charged, subatomic particle.

Enzyme: A protein that can speed up (catalyse) a specific chemical reaction, without being changed or consumed in the process.

Evolution: The process of change over time. In particular, the adaptation of an organism to its environment.

Extinction: The complete elimination of a population or species.

Fenton reaction: A class of reactions, discovered in 1893 by Henry Fenton. The most usual type of Fenton reaction is between iron and hydrogen peroxide, following the equations:

$$Fe^{2+} + H_2O_2 \rightarrow Fe^{3+} + OH^{\cdot} + OH^-$$

$$Fe^{3+} + H_2O_2 \rightarrow Fe^{2+} + OOH^{\cdot} + H^+$$

The reaction converts hydrogen peroxide into hydroxyl and peroxide radicals. In the reactions discussed in this book, vitamin C reacts with iron or copper in cells, to produce hydrogen peroxide.

Folic acid: a water-soluble B-vitamin, found in leafy vegetables (its name comes from the Latin *folium*, from which we also get the word foliage). Folic acid helps in cell reproduction and can prevent anaemia.

Free radical: A molecule or atom with an unpaired electron. Most free radicals are highly reactive; oxidising free radicals are generally damaging to body tissues.

Fructose: Also known as levulose, chemical formula $C_6H_{12}O_6$. A sugar found in most fruits. While fructose is sweeter than glucose, it has a lower glycaemic index.

Gene: The fundamental unit of heredity.

Genome: All the genetic information possessed by an organism, the entire genetic complement.

GI: See Glycaemic Index

Glucose: A simple sugar, chemical formula $C_6H_{12}O_6$, the principal energy source in humans. When people speak of 'blood sugar', they are speaking of blood glucose levels.

Glycaemic index (GI): A numerical measure of how fast the carbohydrate content of a food raises blood sugar levels. The quicker the blood glucose level rises, the higher the glycaemic index. Cooked potatoes, for example, have a very high glycaemic index, while oats and rice have lower GIs. Juices and pulps have higher GIs than whole, solid fruits.

Growth: an increase in tissue size or cell number, especially when cell division exceeds cell death.

Haem: a complex organic pigment, containing iron and other atoms, to which oxygen binds.

Haemoglobin: the pigment in red blood cells. It binds with oxygen in the lungs, transports it around the body and releases it to cells that need it.

Helicobacter pylori: A bacterium that lives in the stomach and duodenum, which causes stomach ulcers and gastritis. The link between the bacterium and these diseases was first shown in 1979, but it was not until the mid-1990s that it became accepted among the medical community as a whole.

Herbivore: An animal that eats only plant matter, as opposed to carnivores (which eat only meat) and omnivores (which eat both).

Herceptin: The trade name for Trastuzumab, a drug created by the biotech company, Genentech. This drug has proved controversial, due to its public perception as a 'breast cancer wonder drug', high costs, and marginal efficacy.

Hydrogen peroxide: A chemical substance (H_2O_2). Normally, a clear, viscous liquid, with strong oxidising properties.

Iron: A metal that is necessary for many processes in the body. Iron drives Fenton reactions (*q.v.*), and acts with vitamin C and lipoic acid to kill cancer cells.

Isothiocyanates: A group of chemicals, such as mustard oil, found in cruciferous plants, including cabbage. These have been shown to have a strong effect in inhibiting carcinogenesis.

Lactose: A sugar found in milk; chemical formula $C_{12}H_{22}O_{11}$. Digesting this sugar requires an enzyme, lactase, which is not present in some people after childhood.

Laetrile: A substance derived from amygdalin; claimed to be an anticancer agent.

Lecithin: A phospholipid (type of fat) found in egg yolk and soy beans, among other sources.

Liposomal vitamin C: A new form of vitamin C. The vitamin is contained within microscopic balls of lecithin (liposomes). Our recent experiments have shown that this form of vitamin C produces high blood plasma levels with high doses (plasma levels $>= 400$ µM/L can be sustained).

Lymphatic system: A secondary circulatory system within the body, an essential part of the human immune system.

Lymphoma: Any of a variety of types of cancer that attack the cells of the lymphatic system, especially lymphocytes (white blood cells). Lymphomas account for about five percent of all cancers.

Malignant: Cells or tumours that grow in an uncontrolled fashion. Such growth may spread into nearby tissue, or may reach distant sites, via the bloodstream or lymphatic system.

Metastases: Secondary tumours; the spread of cancer from one part of the body to another, typically by way of the lymphatic system or bloodstream.

Microevolution: Subspecies-level evolutionary changes, which include adaptation to local environments.

Micronutrient: A term sometimes used for nutrients that are only needed in small amounts in the diet. This term can be inaccurate if applied to substances, like vitamin C, which are needed in far larger amounts than often thought.

Motexafin gadolinium: A drug (commercially name Xcytrin) which drives redox cycles in cancer cells, in a similar way to vitamin K3. This drug works on similar principles to several of the nutritional treatments described in this book, but, unlike them, is patentable.

Mutation: A change (in the number, arrangement or nucleotide sequence) in DNA coding; a permanent, heritable change in a gene or chromosome structure.

Niacin: The chemical $C_6H_5NO_2$, one of several related substances grouped under the label vitamin B3.

Nucleus: An organelle (or subcellular body) that contains most of the cell's genetic material. The nucleus controls chemical reactions within the cell, and stores genetic information (DNA) needed for cellular division

Oncogene: A gene (such as ras) that facilitates the development of cancer, typically by regulating cell growth.

Orthomolecular medicine: The use of natural dietary substances for good health and the treatment of disease, with emphasis on individual variability.

Osteoporosis: A disease in which the mineral density of bones becomes significantly lower, making them more susceptible to fracture.

Oxidation: The addition of oxygen, removal of hydrogen, or removal of electrons from a molecule; the opposite of reduction.

Pharmacological: Relating to pharmacology – the study of how substances interact with organisms to produce a change in function. In the context of this book, a pharmacological dose of a substance is one that is expected to produce a change in physiology, as opposed to a nutritional dose, which would maintain current health.

Phytonutrients: Also known as phytochemicals, this term applies to chemicals found in plants which, while not essential like vitamins, nevertheless have a beneficial effect on health. Many are antioxidants, and often give plants a bright colour, e.g. yellow corn or red tomatoes.

Population control: Limiting the growth of a population, e.g. by changing the proportion of dividing to dying cells.

Protein: Major structural component of body tissue; necessary for cellular growth and repair. Enzymes are proteins.

Quinone: A member of a class of aromatic yellow compounds, including several that are biologically important as coenzymes or vitamins.

Radiotherapy: Use of radiation as a treatment for cancer.

Ras: An oncogene, originally isolated from rat sarcoma virus.

RDA: Recommended Dietary Allowance – government-suggested levels of nutrients. In many cases, these are close to the minimum needed to prevent symptoms of deficiency diseases, and are lower than the optimum level for health. For this reason, some nutritionists suggest that these letters should stand for Ridiculous Dietary Allowance.

Redox: Abbreviation of REDuction-OXidation, which occur together in biochemical reactions.

Redox cycle: Repeated oxidation and reduction of a molecule or group of molecules.

Redox therapy: The use of substances which have oxidising or reducing effects to treat diseases.

Reduction: The opposite of oxidation – the removal of oxygen, addition of hydrogen, or addition of electrons to a molecule.

Risk: Combination of the frequency, or probability, of occurrence and the consequence of a specific, dangerous event.

Sarcoma: A cancer of connective or supportive tissue, such as bone, cartilage, fat or muscle.

Selection pressure: When a number of individuals in a population are competing for access to a finite resource, leading to the death of those least able to gain the resource, the individuals are said to be under 'selection pressure'. The same idea is known popularly as 'survival of the fittest'.

Species: The basic unit of biological classification; a group of organisms with characteristics that distinguish them from other organisms. If they reproduce sexually, individuals within the same species produce viable, fertile offspring.

Stem cell: A cell from which other types of cells can develop.

Tumour: An abnormal tissue growth, or cancerous lump, which may be benign or malignant.

Tumour suppressor gene: A repressor gene that inhibits cancer growth.

Turmeric: See curcumin.

Virus: A tiny organism, consisting of protein and DNA or RNA, which multiples within cells and can cause disease.

Vitamin: An essential, low molecular weight organic compound, required for normal growth and metabolic processes. Lack of one or more vitamins in the diet results in deficiency disease.

White blood cell: Cells within the bloodstream, whose function is to fight infections. They are a major part of the immune system.

X-ray: High energy electromagnetic radiation of very short wavelength; used in medical diagnostics and treatment.

Zinc: A metallic element, found in animal proteins and grains, necessary for a variety of biological processes.

About the authors

Hilary Roberts' PhD research in Nutrition was carried out in the Department of Child Health, at the University of Manchester. Steve Hickey has a PhD in Medical Biophysics from the University of Manchester and is a faculty member at Staffordshire and Manchester Metropolitan Universities. Previous books by the authors include *Ascorbate: The Science of Vitamin C, Ridiculous Dietary allowance and Cancer: Nutrition and Survival.*

The cover image is an anaplastic (microcellular, oat cell) carcinoma of the lung. This image was taken in the Department of Clinical Pathomorphology and Cytology in the Medical University, Lodz, Poland.